Chinese Herbal Medicine

By

C. P. Li, M. D.

THE BOOK TREE

San Diego, California

First published 1974
John E. Fogarty International Center for
Advanced Study in Health Sciences
U.S. Dept. of Health, Education and Welfare

ISBN 1-58509-219-3

Cover layout & design
Lee Berube

Printed on Acid-Free Paper
in the United States of America

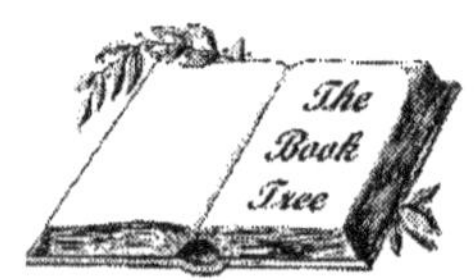

Published by
The Book Tree
P O Box 16476
San Diego, CA 92176
www.thebooktree.com
We provide fascinating and educational products to help awaken the public to new ideas and information that would not be available otherwise.
Call 1 (800) 700-8733 for our ***FREE BOOK TREE CATALOG.***

FOREWARD

The Chinese were the first to invent so many things that it boggles the mind, and their medicine is no exception. Much of their herbal remedies have been proven to work, but have still not been adopted into Western medicine to any large or accepted degree, as evidenced by the information in the Preface.

Most of the herbal medicines described in this volume are from ancient sources. They were developed at a time when the Chinese were fiercely protective of foreigners and chose to remain isolated from the world. Therefore, many valuable innovations and medical practices were never shared with other countries.

This book was written by a research scientist, so is presented in a very technical format. It is ideal for the serious medical researcher or student, as well those wishing to explore alternative medical treatments. Some of the plants involved can only be found in China, but it is possible that those deemed safe by the U.S. government, before and after the book's original publication, could be available. In larger cities there exists Chinese communities that have health and herb shops used by those in the community who could readily acquire such healing items in China, but would otherwise be unable to procure them here. Such places are often helpful to those who wish alternative treatments.

We do not recommend these treatments, as we are not in the business of doing so. We are simply reproducing this book for educational purposes—to allow people to make choices on their own that hold the potential to make a positive difference, and to allow researchers to explore the possibilities of using these herbal remedies in a more complete way.

This book was first published by the U.S. Department of Health, Education, and Welfare in 1974, specifically by the John E. Fogarty International Center for Advanced Study in the Health Sciences. We therefore believe that the information contained herein is of the highest scientific caliber and contains accurate test data.

Paul Tice

Other Publications of the Geographic Health Studies Project
JOHN E. FOGARTY INTERNATIONAL CENTER
for
ADVANCED STUDY IN THE HEALTH SCIENCES

China Health Studies

Medicine and Public Health in the People's Republic of China

Topics of Study Interest in Medicine and Public Health in the People's Republic of China: Report of a Planning Meeting

A Bibliography of Chinese Sources on Medicine and Public Health in the People's Republic of China: 1960-1970

Anticancer Agents Recently Developed in the People's Republic of China - A Review

Prevention and Treatment of Common Eye Diseases*

Neurology - Psychiatry in the People's Republic of China*

Standard Surgical Techniques, Illustrated*

A Barefoot Doctor's Manual*

China Medicine As We Saw It

*Translations of Chinese documents, produced in limited quantities only.

PREFACE

The Fogarty International Center Center initiated in 1969 a series of health studies designed to provide comparative knowledge of the health systems of other countries.

In view of the vast differences in the political, economic and social structure between the United States and the Soviet Union, the Center selected the Soviet health system as its first field of study. To date, 12 publications have resulted.

In 1970, the Center enlarged its study program to include an examination of the health system of the People's Republic of China and its first publication, Medicine and Public Health in the People's Republic of China, has received wide distribution. Additional publications, as well as translations of existing Chinese material, are found on page ii of this document.

Dr. C. P. Li, a distinguished Chinese-born scientist and author of Anticancer Agents Recently Developed in the People's Republic of China, was invited to study and document the ancient, and apparently successful, practices of the Chinese utilizing medicinal herbs. Dr. Li received approval from the People's Republic of China to examine the use and research on herbs by the medical community in China.

The Fogarty International Center does not encourage the use of or experimentation with the herbs mentioned in this document. Rather, it is our hope that the information provided will assist in further scientific investigation and understanding of the subject. A cautionary note should be called to the attention of the reader. Many herbal preparations have irregular modes of entry and distribution in the United States which do not follow the regulatory procedures of the Food and Drug Administration and the U.S. Customs Service, which deny entry of unproven drugs. For example, on June 1, 1974, the Food and Drug Administration issued a warning against the unauthorized use of imported Chinese herbal medications that contain powerful and potentially dangerous ingredients such as phenylbutazone and aminopyrine. Use of these drugs has caused the death of one person and the hospitalization of others.

Although this document is published by an agency of the United States Government, it does not necessarily represent the views of the National Institutes of Health, the Department of Health, Education, and Welfare or any other agency of the Federal Government.

Any inquiries concerning this publication should be directed to Dr. Joseph R. Quinn, Geographic Health Studies Program, Fogarty International Center, National Institutes of Health, Bethesda, Maryland 20014.

Milo D. Leavitt, Jr., M.D.
Director
Fogarty International Center

TABLE OF CONTENTS

Appendix

Pharmacognosy of Individual Herbs Discussed in this Monograph

PART 1

TRADITIONAL HERBAL MEDICINE - AN OVERVIEW

PART 1

TRADITIONAL HERBAL MEDICINE - AN OVERVIEW

1. Introduction and historical background.

The usefulness of certain herbs and other flora as healing agents has been known for thousands of years. Knowledge concerning their medicinal properties and instructions as to their correct application have been handed down from one generation to the next. In the course of time, a substantial body of folk medicine was developed throughout the world. Today, we can count many valuable drugs derived from ancient remedies, such as digitalis, quinine and atropine (2). For centuries, the natives of India chewed snakeroot (Rauwolfia serpentina) for its calming effect. More recently, it was found that snakeroot contains reserpine, now widely recognized as a tranquilizer. The catharantus plant which grows in profusion in Madagascar and the Philippines once was believed to be associated with hypoglycemia but when its constituents were isolated in a modern scientific laboratory, the plant was found to contain the antileukemic agents vincristine and vinblastine (2).

Chinese traditional medicine, however, is not precisely in the category of folk medicine. It is a well-organized system of medical knowledge based on observations, experiments, and clinical trials, all duly recorded, and a body of theory that evolved from the findings. It is not based on empirical experience alone but is a system developed in the distant past by individual scholars and government institutions. Admittedly, not all the theories are grounded on scientific principles, but the effectiveness of a number of the old remedies has been verified by modern science. Acupuncture, for example, is a technique in which the numerous points were elaborated over a period of 2,000 years. And many of the principles first advanced centuries ago have now been confirmed by modern science. Thus, it has become evident that we cannot write off Chinese traditional medicine.

Acupuncture is only one branch of Chinese traditional medicine. The time-honored practice of herbal medicine covers a much larger field and is much more common. The importance of herbal medicine is not limited to the biological activity of each individual herb. Some knowledge of the pathological physiology of certain illnesses can be gained through the study of such herbs (see below).

Approximately 2,000 years ago, the Chinese summarized their medical knowledge up to that time in a medical classic called Nei-ching which consisted of 18 volumes with 162 chapters (42). Of course, books written at that time were not very scientific according to present standards but they contained valuable observations. For instance, Nei-ching said that blood flows through the blood vessels in a regular course and that the function of the blood is to distribute nutrition. Shortly after the publication of Nei-ching, the Chinese published a second medical classic, Shen Nung Ben Tsao (a book of materia medica). The second book listed more than three hundred medicines and described their therapeutic properties.

From time to time since then, knowledge about medicinal plants has been expanded. Under the Tang Dynasty, around A.D. 657, the government ordered one of the leading statesmen to revise the book of materia medica. More than 2,000 scholars were engaged on the project and the revised book was published in A.D. 659 (42).

Another revision of the old text on materia medica was undertaken by the famed Li Shih-chen during the Ming Dynasty. Li Shih-chen studied more than 800 reference books, travelled over most of China and interviewed scholars as well as peasants. He collected 1,892 different kinds of medicinal materials, and divided them into 16 classes which he subdivided further into 60 divisions. He devoted 27 years to the preparation of the new book, called Ben Ts'ao Kang Mu, or the Chinese Pharmacopoeia. First published in 1578, the book contains more than 1,000 standard medical prescriptions, many of them still in use at the present time.

In the summer of 1973, the author spent two months in the People's Republic of China and learned that Chinese biomedical scientists have made remarkable advances in the field of traditional herbal medicine during the past 20-25 years. Chinese scientists have developed a number of herbal drugs for the treatment of coronary diseases with encouraging results. These drugs can be administered orally or intravenously, alone or in combination with Western medicine, Chinese clinicians point out. They have successfully treated acute appendicitis using only herbs (see below). Chinese scientists have isolated a number of useful chemical compounds from herbs, determined their formulas, and successfully synthesized some of them (see below).

The recent advances in China in the field of herbal medicine are highlighted in this monograph. The material discussed in these pages comes from a number of different sources. It includes personal observation and information obtained while visiting various Chinese medical facilities, and conversations with medical authorities in Peking, Shanghai and other cities. In addition, the author is the fortunate owner of a motion picture entitled "Chinese Medicinal Herbs" produced by the China Film Distribution and Exhibition Corporation, Peking. The film describes a number of useful herbs that have been studied recently in China. And although it gives neither scientific data nor references, the film does show the progress that has occurred.

Within the past two or three years, the Chinese have published a large number of books on the subject of traditional medicine, including descriptions and data about the medicinal herbs of each province -- nearly every province has published its own separate volume or volumes on pharmacology and pharmacognosy (3,6,10,14,15, 16,17,19,26,27,28,29,30,31,32,40,43,44,45,55,56,57,60,61,62,63,68, 71,76).

In addition, a number of such books have been published in Hong Kong (7,21,23,25,48,69).

Scientific data of great value were provided the author by the Chinese Medical Association which sent him, via air mail, every issue of the Chinese Medical Journal that contained pertinent information. Other important information was obtained through correspondence with Chinese friends active in the field of herbal medicine.

It is regrettable that certain practical considerations limit the scope of the present report, and that a lack of detailed information concerning some herbs places a limitation on the discussion of medicinal herbs. Consequently, the emphasis will be on herbal medicine.

At this point, it is in order to note that the philosophy and principles of present-day Chinese medicine aim at integrating traditional medicine with Western biomedical science to form one body of medical knowledge. This is the trend that is shaping the future of medicine in China. And it is the author's hope that this monograph will prepare Western biomedical scientists to consider the new ideas from China.

But the author believes it important to state at the outset that he does not advocate going back to folk medicine; nor does he wish to encourage people to treat themselves with great-grandmother's remedies. It should be pointed out that some medicinal herbs are especially toxic and reliance on herbs alone could delay the treatment of serious illnesses. Emphatically, thorough investigation is indicated before medicinal herbs can be used safely and effectively by the health professional.

2. In light of recent discoveries, why was the field of traditional herbal medicine not fully explored until a little more than two decades ago?

The answer to the question is as follows:

First, there were many mistakes in the past. During the early half of this century, scientists did study Chinese herbal medicine without finding anything exciting (33,49,50,53) -- except with respect to ephedrine (2). The chief mistake apparently was that research usually started with the chemical components. When the investigators failed to isolate any active principle, they gave up. They failed to realize that it is necessary to test the biological activity first and to prepare the herb according to traditional methods. Another mistake arose from the fact that the scientists usually worked with a single herb, though the benefits of Chinese herbal medicine most frequently result from the combination of herbs.

Second, it was not until 1949 that Chinese scientists, in response to government policy, began to conduct research in herbal medicine.

Finally, it was because since 1949 great advances in scientific knowledge made it possible to solve some of the problems in traditional medicine.

3. Finding the keys to understanding traditional medicine.

The Chinese government opened a large number of training classes in traditional medicine and admitted graduates from standard medical schools -- including the old Peking Union Medical College -- who had several years of clinical or research experience. These Chinese biomedical scientists, trained in both Western and traditional medicine, have been conducting extensive research in the ancient art. They have greatly increased our understanding of traditional medicine. To illustrate: When an old Chinese medical classic says that a certain prescription is good for spleen illness, the Chinese doctors found that no such spleen illness existed and that the treatment had nothing to do with spleen illness. However, when the same prescription was given to patients suffering from gastrointestinal disturbance, beneficial effects sometimes resulted. This, and other work, led to the conclusion that the ancient Chinese ideograph for spleen didn't mean spleen in the modern sense - we think of spleen as an organ but the ancient Chinese ideograph for spleen referred to the entire gastrointestinal system (45).

Similar interpretations were found applicable to the ancient Chinese ideographs for liver, kidney, lung, etc. Thus, the ancient ideograph for the kidney could mean the entire internal secretory system. Certain drugs said to be capable of regulating liver function show therapeutic benefits in certain eye diseases when the drug is administered orally. "Drugs for the lungs" are found to be effective for some skin conditions. All these new interpretations of the ancient medical classics are being studied extensively by various authorities including Dr. Li Bin (45) and her staff at the Tumor Institute of the Chinese Academy of Medical Sciences, Peking. The main concern of Chinese medical scientists is the long, slow process of understanding an ancient art in the light of modern science, rather than with getting Chinese and Western doctors together to share knowledge.

4. The implication of ancient theories for modern medicine.

Chinese traditional medicine is replete with theories. One of the fundamental therapeutic principles is "Fu Chen Pei Ben" which means: When a person is seriously ill, his or her normal physiological function becomes abnormal and his or her vitality (resistance) is reduced. It is then the task of the physician to make the physiology return to normal and to cultivate the vitality or resistance against the invaders -- the harmful agents or stress.

An example of the progress being made toward understanding the old therapeutic methodology involves experimental studies with animals using a number of traditional prescriptions. These prescriptions were shown to be effective in promoting intestinal peristalsis, in increasing the blood flow in the intestines, and in removing toxic materials. The successful animal studies encouraged the clinicians to use these prescriptions in the treatment of acute abdominal conditions in humans, including acute appendicitis (72,73). Selected patients who were treated with these prescriptions got well without surgery. A more detailed description of the use of this therapeutic regimen is given in Part II.

It has been said by some that developing countries such as China must depend more on native herbal medicine because they cannot afford expensive modern medical facilities and techniques. Undoubtedly this was the situation in China during the civil war and in the early years after the establishment of the present government. But the situation has changed significantly. China has organized the mass production of penicillin and streptomycin. These drugs are inexpensive and freely available. Yet Chinese physicians continue to treat acute appendicitis without surgery, using the ancient prescriptions, not for reasons of economy but because the doctors believe that herbal medicine is eminently more effective than any other form of therapy.

5. Collection, processing, storage, classification and administration.

Because of its great size, China has a wide variety of climatic conditions, soil, and terrain. Many varieties of plants are grown throughout the country and up to the present time, more than 2,000 medicinal herbs have been identified and collected (5). The Government of the People's Republic of China encourages not only the collection of old and new herbs but also the extended cultivation of medicinal plants. And today, China is mass-producing many of the important drugs derived from medicinal plants, including ginseng, a herb which is used in the treatment of hypotension and as a tonic in cardiac conditions.

There is variety in the parts of medicinal plants used for therapeutic purposes. In some, the roots are used; in others, it may be the stem, the leaves, the flowers, the fruits, or the whole plant - and since different parts of a given plant mature at different seasons, collecting the medicinal part at the right time requires special attention.

The processing of medicinal plants is directed toward increased efficacy of the drug. Cleaning the product, it has been found, facilitates storage. Proper cleaning methods eliminate or reduce toxicity, thus enhancing the efficacy and safety of the product, and this facilitates the compounding of a prescription.

In general, processing consists of the following steps: Sorting, washing, slicing and drying. Then the processed drugs may be stored in glass jars or wooden cases. The product is kept dry, protected from insects and worms, and exposed at regular intervals to the sun and air. All these processes are carried out by the personnel of Chinese drug stores which, in recent years, have been expanded into factories.

When a physician has written a prescription, it is brought to the drug store where the herbs are measured out into a package. A machine for use in this procedure was devised recently (5). The drugs are weighed according to the Chinese system of measurement. The usual unit is one chien, the equivalent of 3.12 g.

The package containing the drugs is taken home and boiled in a non-metal utensil for a specified length of time in a prescribed amount of water. The purpose of boiling the herbs in water is to provide a specific amount extract which the patient is required to drink. At a later time within a single day, the herbs are boiled once more to provide the second part of the regimen.

PART II

RECENT EXPERIMENTAL STUDIES AND CLINICAL APPLICATION

Part II

RECENT EXPERIMENTAL STUDIES AND CLINICAL APPLICATION

In the preceding pages, we have emphasized the extraordinary efforts made by Chinese biomedical scientists during the past 20-25 years to modernize traditional herbal medicine. These efforts are reflected most vividly in the number and variety of experimental studies and new clinical applications of the traditional remedies.*

However, before proceeding, it should be noted that the description of the biological activity of certain herbs discussed in this section may not in every instance tally with the information to be found in the Appendix to this monograph. This is because here we are concerned with the combined effects of several drugs and with more recently acquired data.

Chinese biomedical scientists usually approach the study of medicinal herbs in two steps: First, they collect and identify as many medicinal herbs as possible; next, they analyze the herbs chemically, pharmacologically, and clinically.

In the process of studying the herbs, the scientists may begin by analyzing single agents and then studying the effects of the combination of several agents in compound prescriptions. The isolation of ephedrine (4) was achieved during an analysis of a single agent. At the present time, the Chinese have identified a number of new isolates, some of which are as important as ephedrine. One of these new isolates is anisodamine.

1. Studies on single agents, e.g. anisodamine.

Anisodamine (12,13,24,58) is an alkaloid isolated from the Chinese solancea plant, _Anisodus tanuticus_ (Maxim.) Pascher or _Scopolia tangutica_ Maxim.** Its hydrobromide salt is a white needle-like crystal, easily soluble in water with a melting point of 162-164°C and a specific rotation of D^{18}- 10.4 (H_2O, C 2.24). Its formula (Chart 1) is similar to that of atropine. It has also been synthesized. The isolated natural product is designated as "654" and the synthesized one "654-2". These two products are identical in their pharmacological action as well as in clinical effects.

1.1 Pharmocology

The physiologic disposition of anisodamine in rats and also in men has been reported as follows (12):

*The various herbs discussed here are shown in the Appendix, listed alphabetically according to their scientific names.
**A picture of this herb is not available.

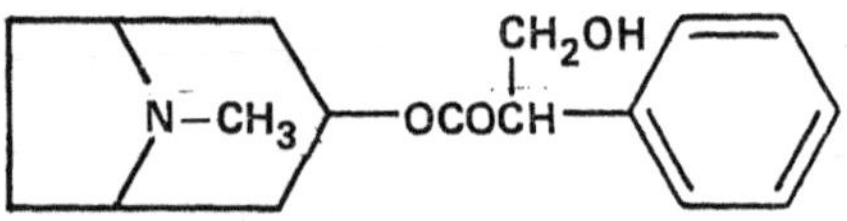

N–CH_3 —OCOCH(—CH_2OH)—

Atropine

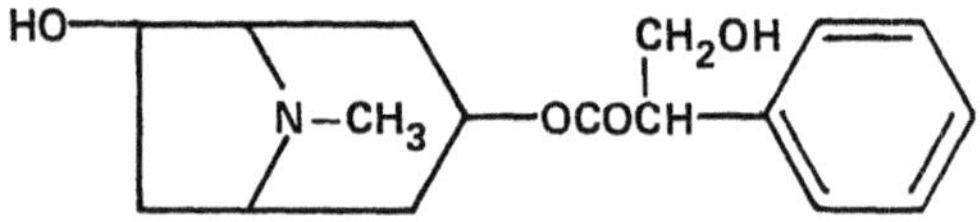

HO— N–CH_3 —OCOCH(—CH_2OH)—

Anisodamine (6(s)-hydroxyhyoscyamine)

Chart 1. Structural formulas of atropine and anisodamine (14)

Highest concentrations of anisodamine were found in the kidneys of rats 15 minutes after an intravenous injection of the drug. The kidney levels fell so rapidly that only one-fifth of the value was obtained 30 minutes after an intravenous injection (Chart 2). At this time interval, the highest drug concentrations were found in the pancreas; moderate concentrations in the lungs, heart, kidneys, spleen and liver; and low concentrations in the brain and plasma. When equal doses of anisodamine and atropine were given to rats intravenously, the concentrations of anisodamine were much higher than those of atropine in the pancreas, whereas the opposite was true in the kidneys (Chart 3). Drug distribution studies were also carried out on autopsy materials from two children with fulminating epidemic meningitis who received anisodamine treatment before death. It seems that higher concentrations could be found in human tissues than in those of healthy rats.

The 24-hour urinary excretions of anisodamine were determined in rats, sick children and healthy volunteers. After an intravenous dose of anisodamine in a rat, the 24-hour urinary excretion of unchanged drug was found to be 38.8 percent of the injected dose as compared with 17.4 percent urinary excretion following the injection of atropine (Chart 4). Two sick children who received anisodamine intravenously excreted 41.7 percent and 49.1 percent of the doses in the 24-hour urine, respectively. The 24-hour urinary excretion of the drug, after intramuscular injections, was found to be 31.6 percent - 48.2 percent in both sick children and healthy subjects.

After intravenous injection of anisodamine in rats, the "half life" of the drug in the body was found to be only 40 minutes, indicating that the drug is either excreted or metabolized (or both) rapidly.

The "half absorption time" of anisodamine in rats given orally was determined to be 3.5 hours. Data obtained from drug excretion studies on healthy men suggest that during the first 4-hour period, anisodamine concentrations in human tissues after an oral dose of 30 mg may be roughly the same as after an intramuscular injection dose of 10 mg.

1.2 Side effects as compared with atropine

The pharmacologic effects of anisodamine on the central and peripheral nervous systems as compared with those of atropine sulfate (13) were tested by three methods: (a) Observation of the antagonistic action in mice against tremorine-induced tremor. (b) The influence of anisodamine on the conditioned avoidance response of rats. (c) The effect on EEG of cats bearing chronic implanted electrodes.

The findings indicated that the action of this alkaloid was 6-20 times weaker than that of atropine. After intraperitoneal injection of anisodamine at the dosage of 20 mg per kg body weight in unanesthetized cats, the arousal behavior usually seen after the injection of 2-3 mg/kg of atropine was scarcely observable.

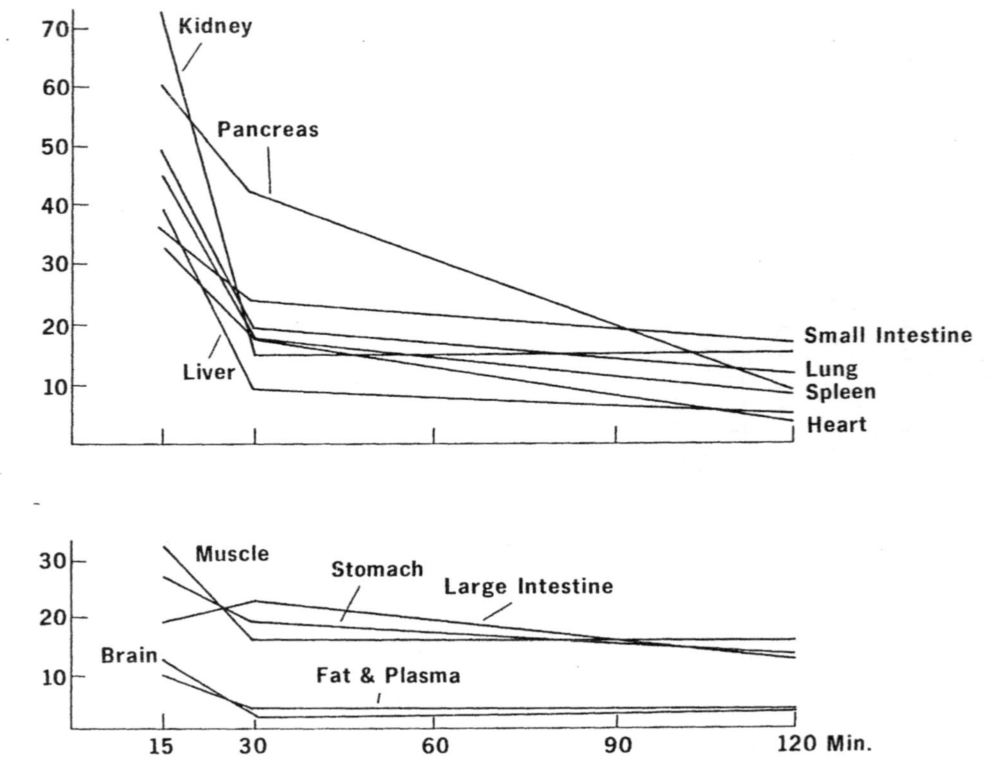

Chart 2. The distribution of drug in the body after intravenous injection of anisodamine 50 mg/kg of body weight of rats (12).

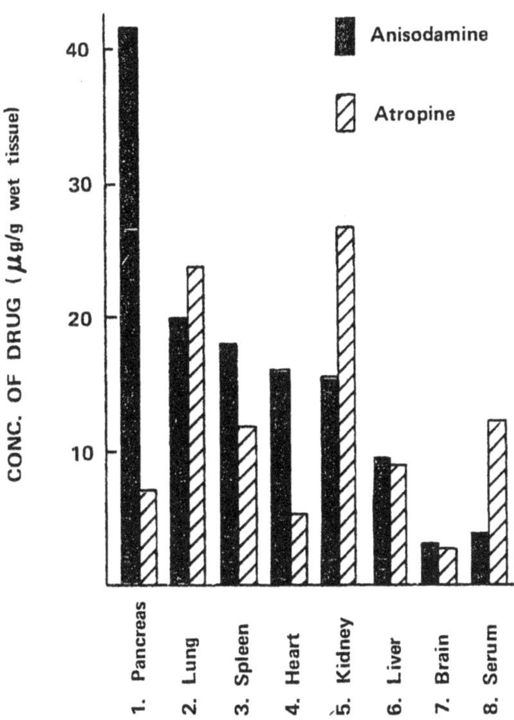

Chart 3. The comparison of drug distribution in the body of rats 30 min. after intravenous injections of anisodamine and atropine, 50 mg/kg of body weight (12).

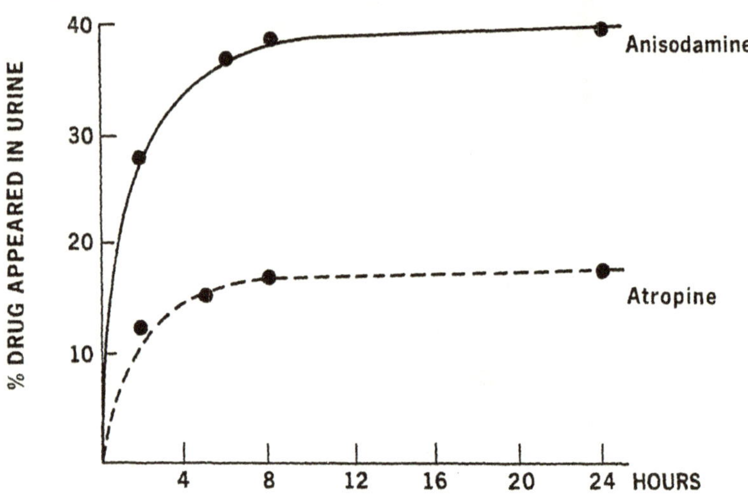

Chart 4. Comparison of Anisodamine and Atropine in urine of rats after intravenous injections of 30 mg/kg of body weight of the respective drug (12).

There was evidence that anisodamine is a new anticholinergic drug with a strong spasmolytic property. The spasm of the isolated small intestine and urinary bladder of rats and cats induced by acetylcholine can be antagonized by the administration of anisodamine and atropine. The tonus of the small intestine, in situ, of cats and rabbits could also be decreased. Anisodamine was capable of inhibiting the decrease in blood pressure that followed acetylcholine administration. These actions of the alkaloid were of the same order as those of atropine.

Anisodamine and atropine in the same dosage (i.p. 4, 7 and 12 mg/kg) will antagonize the toxic action of certain drugs such as DFP (diisopropylfluorophosphate) and dipterex. This effect can be seen in the elevation of the LD_{50} of the organic phosphorus compounds in mice. Symptoms such as salivation and sweating could be diminished by intraperitoneal injection of either drugs.

However, the inhibitory effect of anisodamine on salivary secretion was less potent than that of atropine. On subcutaneous injection, it showed one-twentieth the activity of atropine. Both anisodamine and atropine dilated the pupils of mice, but the dosage of atropine required was 10 times smaller (Chart 5).

It was postulated, on the basis of the experimental studies, that anisodamine might be a better spasmolytic agent than atropine, by virtue of its milder activity on the salivary glands, the pupils, and the central nervous system. In other words, anisodamine would produce less untoward effects. This, in fact, has been substantiated by clinical studies (58).

1.3 Toxicity of anisodamine

Acute toxicity -- Determination of LD_{50} of anisodamine (13) was carried out in mice, each weighing 18-24 g and all of the same sex. They were divided into five groups, with 10 in each group. Anisodamine of differing concentrations was injected into the mice intraperitoneally. The number of mice that died in 24 hours was recorded. The LD_{50} of atropine was determined by the same method, and administered simultaneously. The LD_{50} for anisodamine was found to be 350 ± 11 mg/kg, and that of atropine was 226 ± 6 mg/kg. The minimum oral lethal dose of anisodamine was 1600 mg/kg, while that of atropine was 700 mg/kg. By intravenous injections, anisodamine killed mice at a concentration of 123 mg/kg, while atropine killed mice at a concentration of 97.7 mg/kg. Anisodamine, therefore, was found to be less toxic than atropine.

Chronic toxicity -- The effects of anisodamine on the liver, kidney, and blood were studied in dogs (13). A dosage of 2 mg/kg was given to each of three dogs through intravenous injections, administered daily for a period of 2 weeks. During the medication period, and for a few days thereafter, the blood NPN and the residual sulfobromophthalein sodium were determined. The latter

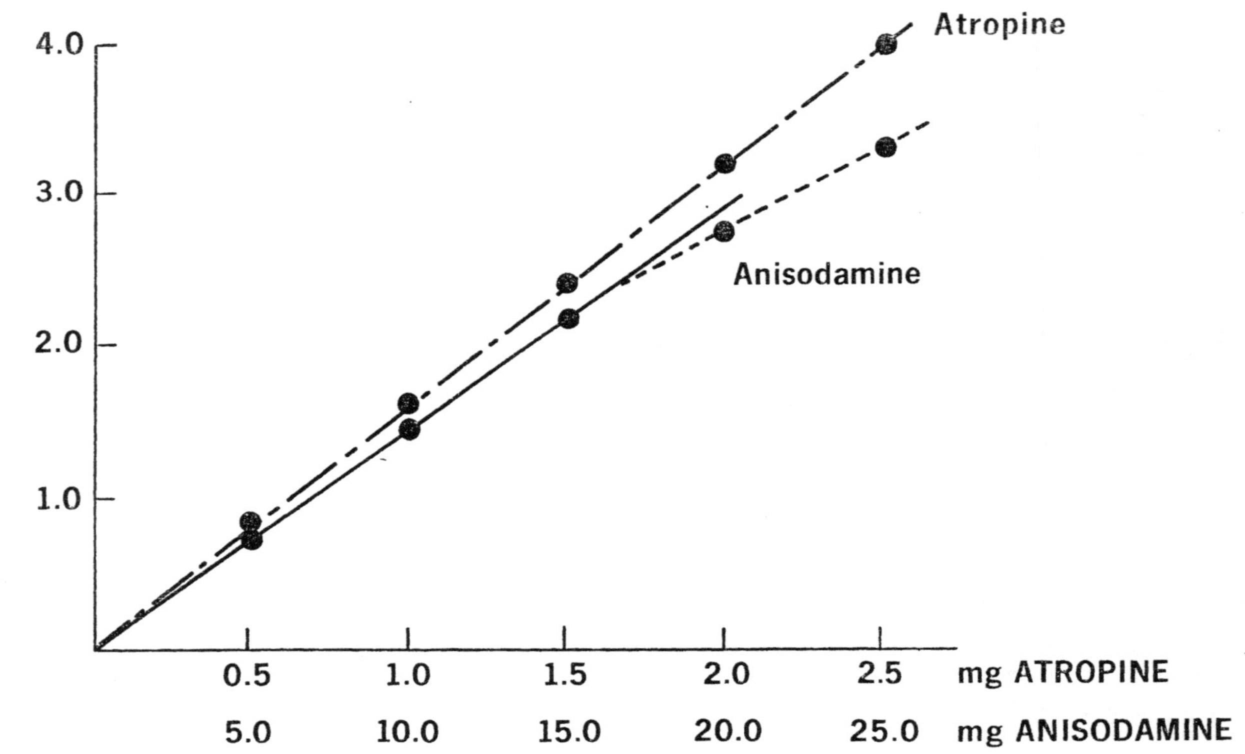

Chart 5. Comparison of effect of atropine and anisodamine on the pupil dilation of mice (12).

also was injected intravenously and tested 45 minutes afterwards. The results indicated that amisodamine has no effects on the liver, kidney, and blood. During the entire medication period, the dogs appeared healthy, active, and with normal appetites.

1.4 Clinical studies -- Effects on diseases of acute microcirculatory disturbances

Since 1965, the Chinese biomedical scientists at Peking have used anisodamine in the treatment of fulminant epidemic meningitis, toxic dysentery, and some similar acute infectious diseases (58). Their clinical results and interpretations are as follows:

Based on the observation of the nailfold microcirculation, funduscopic examinations and clinical practice, it was found that acute microcirculatory disturbances caused by spasm of the arterioles are the chief changes in the early incipient stage of acute infections such as fulminant epidemic meningitis, toxic bacillary dysentery, septic shock, severe lobar pneumonia, and hemorrhagic enteritis; these disturbances are the basis on which serious signs and symptoms of the diseases develop. Variations in microcirculatory disturbances in different parts of the body lead to the formation of different types of clinical manifestations. Cases with coma, convulsions and acute respiratory failure, following severe cerebral anoxia due to disturbances of the cerebral microcirculation, are classified as the cerebral microcirculatory disturbance type (the cerebral type), whereas cases with shock secondary to stasis of blood in the viscera due to disturbances in the visceral microcirculation, as well as purpuric skin lesions, are classified as the dermo-visceral microcirculatory disturbance type (the dermo-visceral type). An additional form is derived from these, namely, the pulmonary microcirculatory disturbance type (the pulmonary type) which occurs comparatively late in an illness. Thus, it is suggested that diseases such as those mentioned above be designated as diseases of acute microcirculatory disturbances.

Pharmacologically, anisodamine is a cholinergic blocking agent capable of antagonizing the spasm of the arterioles caused by acetylcholine, catecholamine and 5-hydroxytryptamine. It is an effective drug for dilating the arterioles and improving the microcirculation. With its use, a number of diseases with acute microcirculatory disturbances have been treated successfully. In 380 cases of fulminant epidemic meningitis, 412 cases of toxic bacillary dysentery and 141 cases of septic shock treated between April, 1965 and December, 1971, using anisodamine in conjunction with other therapeutic measures, the death rate was lowered to 12.4 percent, 0.5 percent, and 12.7 percent respectively. In 48 cases of hemorrhagic enteritis treated by the same method in the period from June, 1965 to August, 1971, the death rate was reduced to 4.2 percent. In 14 cases of severe lobar pneumonia so treated from July, 1965 to December, 1971, not a single death occurred.

This experience serves to show that application of the theory of microcirculatory disturbances offers a new approach to the diagnosis and treatment of a variety of diseases.

1.5 Treatment of severe toxic bacillary dysentery

Good results were obtained at a hospital in Loyang (Central China) (24), in the combined treatment of 23 cases of severe toxic bacillary dysentery with anisodamine (or its synthetic equivalent -- 654-2) as the mainstay. Twelve patients were male and 11 female, aged 1.5-76 years. Eleven cases were in the early stage of the disease and 12 cases in the late stage.

The combined treatment was individualized according to the condition of each patient. It included oxygen inhalation, appropriate antibiotics, hydrocortisone (except in individual cases with mild symptoms), fluid infusion and lowering of temperature by physical measures or medication. Anisodamine was used in all cases to correct microcirculatory disturbances during the process of the disease and given once every 5-15 minutes intravenously or intramuscularly in doses of 0.5-2 mg/kg. This therapy was maintained until the blood pressure was stabilized, facial color returned and the extremities warmed up, and then was gradually discontinued or stopped while a close watch was kept.

Of the 23 patients, all except one were cured. Ten were early stage cases hospitalized 3-15 days, averaging five days; 12 were late stage cases hospitalized 5-28 days, averaging 10.5 days. The fatal case was in the early stage of circulatory failure when admitted, but the patient died of cerebral edema and respiratory failure because the initial doses of anisodamine were insufficient to correct circulatory failure.

Anisodamine has fewer side-effects than atropine, but if inappropriately used, toxic effects similar to those of atropine may appear. In 12 cases, anisodamine caused dryness of the mouth, abdominal distension, restlessness or retention of urine, of which all improved following symptomatic treatment. No prolonged sequelae were observed.

The pathophysiologic processes of microcirculatory disturbances developing during certain stages of toxic bacillary dysentery have been mentioned. Experience has shown that anisodamine is effective in improving microcirculatory blood perfusion and correcting shock, but to ensure better therapeutic results as well as to reduce side-effects, it should be used in combination with other measures and its dose adjusted promptly according to the overall condition of the patient.

2. Studies on compound prescriptions.

2.1 Liu wei di huang tang (decoction of Rehmannia with six components) (34,39,41,69). This is a traditional prescription used for various kidney diseases including those with hypertension. The Chinese biomedical scientists (75) carried out experimental studies with this prescription and found that it has a marked hypotensive effect on experimental renal hypertension in rats. Some of the results are presented here:

The prescription consists of the following ingredients:

"Di-huang" (Rehmannia glutinosa L., steamed root)	25 g
"San-chu-yu" (Fruit of Cornus officinalis S. et Z.)	12.5 g
"San-yao" (Dioscorea batatas Dcne., root)	12.5 g
"Mau-dan-pi" (Paeonia suffruticosa A., root bark)	9.4 g
"Che-shi" (Alisma plantago-aquatica L. var. orientale Sarn, tuber)	9.4 g
"Fu-lin" (Poria cocos (Schw.) Wolf)	9.4 g

In a series of experiments, a large number of male rats (close to 100 animals for each experiment), 2-3 months old, were operated on and both kidneys were partially ligated or one kidney was ligated and the other removed. The blood pressure of the rats rose sharply within 2-3 weeks after the operation and remained steady at high levels. The rats were divided at random into two groups, one for control and the other for treatments. At the end of the third or fourth week, the decoction at a certain calculated dosage per body weight was given to each rat via a stomach tube once daily.

Renal function test was carried out in both groups just before drug treatment and repeated once or twice 4-8 weeks later. It was performed as follows: Nine microcuries of carrier free I^{131}-Urokon was dissolved in 0.25 ml of normal saline and injected rapidly (within 5-10 seconds) into a leg vein. At the end of 1, 2, 3, 10, 30, and 60 minutes after the injection, blood samples were taken from the tail. 0.10 ml of each sample, together with a few drops of distilled water, were uniformly plated on to filter paper in an aluminum planchet. After drying, the samples were counted by a mica window G-M counter (probable errors less than 5 percent). For each rat, the peak value of the specific activity (counts per minute per 0.1 ml blood) was usually found among the first three of the six samples. The relative specific activity of the 10, 30, and 60 minute samples was then calculated to represent the renal function, taking the peak specific activity of the same rat as 100 percent (Table 1).

The relative specific activity of the 10, 30, and 60 minute blood samples of the hypertensive rats (operated) was significantly higher than that of the normal animals (Table 1). This means that renal function was impaired in the operated animals.

After treatment the renal function greatly improved, as shown in the decrease in specific activity (Table 2). The improvement was not due to any spontaneous improvement of the disease, since in the operated but untreated group the relative specific activity did not show significant changes during the same intervals.

As shown in Table 3, the blood pressure of the hypertensive rats was also reduced after the administration of liu wei di huang tang. Besides these changes, the mortality of the treated group was lower than that of the untreated controls (Table 4).

The data show that liu wei di huang tang can really improve the kidney function of rats with renal hypertension, even when no normal kidney has been preserved. Although the improvement is only partial, it is statistically significant. Therefore, it may be concluded that liu wei di huang tang can actually act upon the ligated kidneys to improve their function and may be used clinically.

The drug's effect on the blood pressure is progressive over a period of 8 weeks. Since the same prescription does not reduce the blood pressure of normal rats or rats with adrenocortical hypertension induced by a modified operation of Skelton (64), it is reasonable to suppose that the hypotensive effect of the drug is intimately related to its favorable action on the renal function.

However, there is an additional possibility. It is generally believed that if there is no significant renal sclerosis, the impairment of kidney function in hypertension (including renal hypertension) is mainly caused by decreased renal blood flow, which in turn leads to functional disturbances of the glomeruli and tubules. Since in the above-mentioned experiments postmortem examination of the hypertensive rats (operated) revealed no perceptible renal sclerosis, it is quite possible that liu wei di huang tang is also able to increase the renal blood flow, directly or indirectly.

In conclusion, therefore, it can be said that liu wei di huang tang has been shown to increase the blood circulation of the kidney and/or stimulate the secretory function of the renal tubules.

2.2 Ta cheng chi tang and other related prescriptions

There are a number of traditional prescriptions which have proven effective in the treatment of acute abdominal conditions, including acute appendicitis (72). The Chinese biomedical scientists carried out extensive experimental studies on the pharmacological activities of these prescriptions. Some of these prescriptions and their constituents are listed below:

TABLE 1

COMPARISON OF THE KIDNEY FUNCTION OF RENAL HYPERTENSIVE RATS AND NORMAL RATS (75)

Time of collection of samples (Min. after injection)	Relative specific activity of blood				Remark
	Normal		Hypertensive		
	Rats	$\bar{X} \pm$ S.E.	Rats	$\bar{X} \pm$ S.E.*	
10	16	42.8 ±4.44	30	79.1±3.70	t=19.4 $p<0.01$
30	17	13.0 ±1.35	28	48.2±3.10	t= 8.77 $p<0.01$
60	16	4.95±1.10	32	35.7±3.30	t= 7.02 $p<0.01$

*S.E. = specific activity, see text

TABLE 2

THE EFFECT OF LIU WEI DI HUANG TANG ON THE KIDNEY FUNCTION OF RENAL HYPERTENSIVE RATS (75)

Time of collection of samples (Min. after injection)	Relative specific activity of blood				Remark
	Before treatment		After treatment		
	Rats	X±S.E.	Rats	X±S.E.	
10	23	82.4 ± 4.13	23	62.7 ± 4.16	t=3.20 p 0.01
30	25	54.0 ± 4.03	21	38.3 + 2.80	t=3.26 p.0.01
60	25	38.3 + 3.57	25	13.7 ± 1.62	t=5.00 p.0.01

TABLE 3

EFFECT OF LIU WEI DI HUANG TANG ON THE BLOOD PRESSURE OF RENAL HYPERTENSIVE RATS (OPERATED) (75)

Time of measurement	Untreated		Treated	
	Rats	Mean B.P. (mm Hg)	Rats	Mean B.P. (mm Hg)
Before operation	23	109	21	108
2-4 weeks after operation:	23	132	23	130
After start of drug treatment:				
1 week	23	128	23	115
2 weeks	23	126	23	110
3 weeks	22	130	23	110
4 weeks	21	127	23	104
5 weeks	19	127	20	104
6 weeks	16	126	19	99
7 weeks	13	123	17	97
8 weeks	11	129	17	96

TABLE 4

MORTALITIES OF UNTREATED AND TREATED RATS WITH RENAL HYPERTENSION (75)

Group	Rats	Deaths	Mortality (%)	Remark
Untreated	42	24	57.1	$t=2.25$ $p<0.05$
Treated	22	7	29.1	

Ta cheng chi tang

"Ta-huang" (*Rheum tanguticum* Maxim. et Rgl.)	9.36 g
"Hou-pu" (*Magnolia officinalis* Rehd. et Wils.)	6.24 g
"Chi-shih" (*Citrus aurantium* L.)	9.36 g
"Mu-hsiao" (Sodium sulfate)	9.36 g

Kan sui tang

"Kan-sui" (*Euphorbia sieboldiana* Morr. et Dcne)	0.312 g
"Tao-jen" (*Prunus persica* (L.) Batsch)	9.36 g
"Pe-shou" (*Paeonia lactiflora* Pall)	15.60 g
"Hou-pu" (*Magnolia officinalis* Rehd. et Wils.)	15.60 g
"Sheng-niu-hsi" (*Achyranthes bidentata* Bl.)	9.36 g
"Ta-huang" (*Rheum tanguticum* Maxim. et Rgl.)	15.60 g
"Mu-hsiang" (*Saussurea lappa* Clarke)	9.36 g

San wu pei chi powder

"Pa-tou" (*Croton tiglium* L.)	3.12 g
"Kan-chiang" (*Zingiber officinale* Rosc.)	6.24 g
"Ta-huang" (*Rheum tanguticum* Maxim et Rgl.)	15.60 g

Huo hsueh hua yu tang

"Dan-pi" (*Paeonia suffruticosa* Andr.)	15.60 g
"Pe-shou" (*Paeonia lactiflora* Pall)	15.60 g
"Tang-kuei" (*Angelica sinensis* (Oliv.) Diels)	9.36 g
"Tao-jen" (*Prunus persica* (L.) Batsch)	9.36 g
"Hung-hua" (*Carthamus tinctorius* L.)	9.36 g

Lan wei ching chieh tang *

"Chin-ning-hua" (*Lonicera japonica* Thunb.)	31.20 g
"Pu-kung-yin" (*Taraxacum mongolicum* Hand.-Mazz.)	31.20 g
"Ta-huang" (*Rheum tanguticum* Maxim et Rgl.)	15.60 g
"Dan-pi" (*Paeonia suffruticosa* Andr.)	15.60 g
"Chuan-lien-tze" (*Melia toosendan* Sieb. et Zucc.)	9.36 g
"Tung-kua-jen" (*Benincasa hispida* (Thunb.) Cogn.)	12.48 g

All the preparations have the effect of promoting intestinal peristalsis in mice (Chart 6).

Ta cheng chi tang probably acts directly on the intestinal musculature. This is evidenced by the fact that cervical vagotomy and bilateral adrenalectomy do not interfere with its effect on intestinal contraction in mice and that atropine, hexamethonine bromide and dicaine have no influence on isolated segments of the

*This prescription was recently designed at the Nan-Kai Hospital, Tientsin.

intestine of guinea pigs. The drug also has the effect of reducing intussusception (Table 5) when given orally but shows no effect when given intravenously. Further subcutaneous injections of the decoction into guinea pigs limit the spread of the dyestuff within the skin, inhibit the activity of hyaluronidase and lower the volume of indigo carmine transferred from the blood to the peritoneal cavity.

Ta cheng chi tang combined with huo hsueh hua yu tang promotes circulation of the isolated segment of a dog's intestine, yielding a mean increase of 70 percent of blood flow as compared with the controls. These drugs can in addition inhibit or minimize the elevation of capillary permeability of the intestinal wall resulting from histamine and Co^{60} irradiation.

Lan wei ching chieh tang and huo hsueh hua yu tang possess the ability to inhibit the growth of organisms often seen in the intestinal tract and to detoxify their endotoxins (Table 6).

The Chinese emphasize that in traditional Chinese medicine, theories (physiology, etiology, pathology), methodology (therapeutic principles), prescriptions and drugs constitute a unified whole, and methodology is the pivot. The study of methodology will not only reveal the actions of the drugs, but will also help to throw light on the nature of the disease itself (72).

Since medical theory makes constant progress through practice, the Chinese investigators consider that the examination and employment of drugs that show good empirical results, while not neglecting the quest for a scientific explanation of the success, are of tremendous importance in the integration of traditional Chinese and Western medicine.

3. Treatment of acute appendicitis and gallstones.

The treatment of acute appendicitis with herbal medicine is given here as an illustrative example because it offers a challenge to Western medical practice. Contradictory to the principle of Western medicine, laxatives such as rhubarb and "Mu-hsiao"* are freely used. The use of herbs for treating this disease started in the Nan-Kai Hospital in Tientsin and the Tsun I Hospital in Kweichow Province (67,72,73). It was then widely practiced throughout the country. As also mentioned previously, the principle of treatment is to promote peristalsis so as to expel the bacterial and toxic material from the lumen of the appendix, to increase local blood circulation and to inhibit the growth of bacteria and detoxify their toxins. The common ancient prescription for this purpose is Ta cheng chi tang (see section 2.2) or Ta huang mo dan pi tang:

---

*"Mu-hsiao" has been identified as sodium sulfate (4).

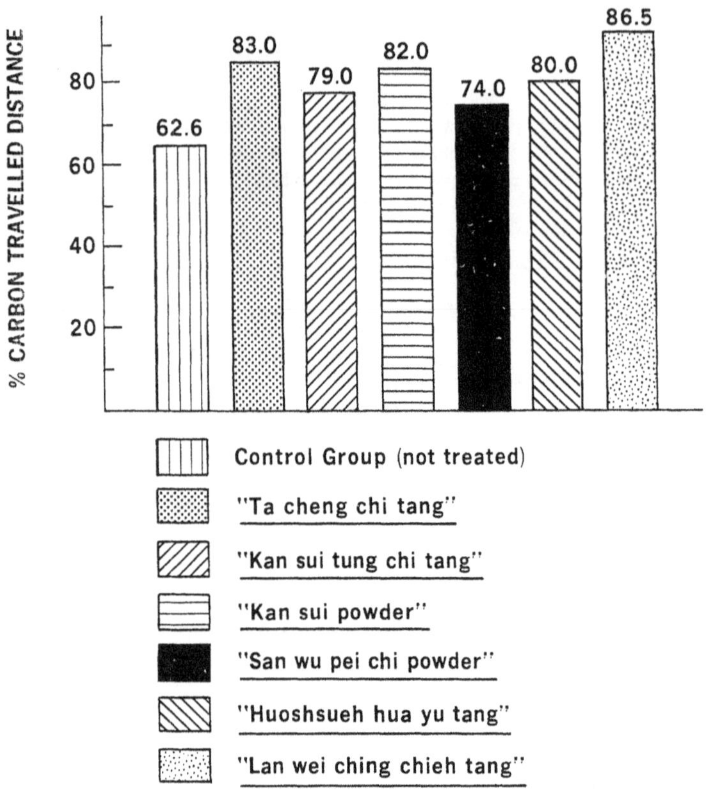

Chart 6. The influence of different prescriptions on intestinal peristalsis (72).

Notes:

1. Twenty mice in each group.

2. A 10 percent suspension of carbon particles together with the concoction of the respective prescription (1:1) were fed by a stomach tube to each group except the controls, which received the carbon suspension without the medicine.

3. All mice were killed 50 minutes after feeding except the group treated with lan wei ching chieh tang, which were killed 60 minutes after feeding.

4. The percent carbon travelled distance was calculated as follows: The entire length from the cardiac entrance of the stomach to the end of the rectum was regarded as the total gastrointestinal distance. The distance from the cardiac entrance of the stomach to the point in the intestine where the carbon particles reached was regarded as the carbon travelled distance. The latter divided by the former x 100 was the percent of carbon travelled distance.

TABLE 5

THE EFFECT OF TA CHENG CHI TANG ON THE REDUCTION OF INTESTINAL INTUSSUSCEPTION IN RABBITS (72)

Experimental group				Control group			
Animal no.	Reduction	*Time	Peristalsis	Animal no.	Reduction	*Time	Peristalsis
12	complete	52'	+	13	none	-	+
15	complete	15'42"	+++	14	none	-	++
18	complete	8'	++	17	complete	40'	+
19	complete	1'49"	++	20	complete	3'	+
21	complete	13'28"	++	24	none	-	+
23	complete	15'	++	26	complete	60	++
25	complete	29"	++	28	none	-	+
27	complete	17'	+++	31	none	-	+
29	complete	12'	+++	32	none	-	++
30	complete	20'2"	+++	33	none	-	++

$P<0.05$

Notes:

1. Ta cheng chi tang was given orally.

2. Intussusception was produced artificially.

3. *Time (after medication) for reduction of intussusception ' = minutes; " = seconds.

4. Peristalsis: + slight; ++ in between + & +++; +++ indicates both transverse and circular muscles showed vigorous and frequent contraction.

TABLE 6

BACTERIA-COUNT IN PERITONEAL FLUID AND THE RESULTS OF BLOOD CULTURE (72)

Date	Experimental Group		Control Group	
	Bacteria Count*	Blood Culture	Bacteria Count*	Blood Culture
Before	-	-	-	-
After 2nd day	10^3	-	10^3	-
3rd day	10^3	-	10^5	-
4th day	0	-	10^5	-
5th day	0	-	0	all rabbits (+)
6th day	0	No. 2 rabbits (+)	0	all rabbits (+)
7th day	10^1	No. 2 rabbits (+)	10^8	all rabbits (+)

Notes:

1. Twelve rabbits were equally divided into two groups. A lethal dose of Escherichia coli was given intraperitoneally to all rabbits.
2. One group was treated intravenously with extracts of herbs (Shuang-hua, Kung-yin, etc.) which are known to be capable of inhibiting bacterial growth and detoxifying bacterial toxins. The other group was not treated for control. The rabbits were killed on the seventh day after infection.
3. All 6 control rabbits developed acute peritonitis within 6 days after infection.
4. Only one of the six treated rabbits showed a mild, localized peritonitis. Another showed a little exudate in the mesentery. All 4 other treated rabbits showed no pathology.
5. The bacteria-count of peritoneal fluid and blood culture are shown in this table.
   * peritoneal bacteria-count per ml.
   0: not enough peritoneal fluid is obtainable for bacteria count; P 0.01.
   - indicates negative.
   + indicates positive.

"Ta-huang" (Rheum tanguticum Maxim. et Rgl.)	12.48
"Dan-pi" (Paeonia suffruticosa Andr.)	9.36
"Tao-jen" (Prunus persica (L.) Batsch)	9.36-15.60
"Mu-hsiao" (Sodium sulfate)	9.36
"Tung-kua-jen" (Benincasa hispida (Thunb.) Cogn.)	15.60-31.20

The following two prescriptions recently designed at Nan-Kai Hospital, Tientsin, also are commonly used:

Lan wei hua yu tang

"Chuan-lien-tze" (Melia toosendan Sieb. et Zucc.)	15.60
"Yan-hi-so" (Corydalis bulbosa DC.)	9.36
"Dan-pi" (Paeonia suffruticosa Andr.)	9.36
"Tao-jen" (Prunus persica (L.) Batsch)	9.36
"Chin-ning-hua" (Lonicera japonica Thunb.)	15.60
"Mu-hsiang" (Saussurea lappa Clarke)	9.36
"Ta-huang" (Rheum tanguticum Maxim. et Rgl.)	9.36
"Ta-hsueh-teng" (Sargentodoxa cuneata (Oliv.) Rehd. et Wils.)	15.60

Lan wei ching chieh tang (modified)

"Chin-ning-hua" (Lonicera japonica Thunb.)	62.40
"Kung-yin" (Taraxacum mongolicum Hand.-Mazz.)	62.40
"Dan-pi" (Paeonia suffruticosa Andr.)	15.60
"Ta-huang" (Rheum tanguticum Maxim. et Rgl.)	24.96-31.20
"Chuan-lien-tze" (Melia toosendan Sieb. et Zucc.)	31.20
"Pe-shou" (Paeonia lactiflora Pall)	12.48
"Tung-kua-jen" (Benincasa hispida (Thunb.) Cogn.)	15.60
"Mu-hsiang" (Saussurea lappa Clarke)	9.36
"Kan-tsao" (Glycyrrhiza uralensis Fisch.)	9.36

A single agent, "Pe-hua-she-shih-tsao" (Oldenlandia diffusa Roxb.) has recently been found almost as effective as the compound prescriptions (41).

In the above-mentioned three compound prescriptions, the laxative, rhubarb, is used among other herbs to ensure free passage of the toxic bacterial mass from the lumen of the appendix. In severe cases, the patient is given enough rhubarb to effect four bowel movements a day with soft stools. The treatment is often accompanied by acupuncture to relieve pain or for other purposes. On one series of 57 cases reported by a hospital in Sian (67), 93.4 percent patients got well in a few days without operation and went back to their normal work. In chronic cases, relapse often occurred after the treatment and where surgery was performed for such cases, "fecal stones" were found inside the appendix, apparently not expelled by medication.

The following case (67) is reported:

Patient Wang, age 55, admitted November 24, 1971. Diagnosis: Acute appendicitis, ruptured, with spreading peritonitis and paralytic intestinal obstruction. Temperature 39.8°C. Leucocytes: 14,200, with 90 percent neutrophiles. All abdominal muscles tense, with tenderness and abdominal distention. Peristalsis not detectable. The patient was given orally the standard Ta cheng chi tang (a mixture of 8 kinds of medicinal substances including sodium sulfate) for 2 days. Intestinal obstruction was then relieved. Treatment was changed to Lan wei ching chieh tang (containing rhubarb). The patient completely recovered without operation or other medication. Discharged on December 13, 1971, he returned to his regular work.

A certain percentage of gallstones cases were effectively treated with herbal medicine without operation (5,34,41,73). The principle is to induce peristalsis of the gallbladder so as to expel the stone. Various prescriptions were used for this purpose; two of them are mentioned below as examples.

Nan-Kai Hospital prescription. Chief ingredients are:

"Chia-hu" (Bupleurum chinense DC.)	9.36
"Pan-hsia" (Pinellia ternata Breit)	9.36
"Mu-hsiang" (Saussurea lappa Clarke)	9.36
"Yu-chin" (Curcuma aromatica Salisb.)	9.36
"Ta-huang" (Rheum tanguticum Maxim. et Rgl.)	9.36

Stone Expelling Mixture No. 5:

"Chin-chien-tsao" (Lysimachia Christinae Hance)	3.12
"Mu-hsiang" (Saussurea lappa Clarke)	9.36
"Chi-kou" (Citrus aurantium L.)	9.36
"Huang-chen" (Scutellaria baicalensis Georgi)	9.36
"Chuan-lien-tze" (Melia toosendan Sieb. et Zucc.)	9.36
"Ta-huang" (Rheum tanguticum Maxim. et Rgl.)	6.24

After the patient has taken the medicine, the secretion of bile is increased and the gallbladder is distended. The patient usually feels distention of the abdomen with pain. Fried eggs are then fed to the patient in order to increase the flow of bile into the intestine. At the same time, acupuncture is used to regulate the physiological function, so that the gallbladder contracts and expels the stone into the intestine. In one such case successfully treated, the author saw the 1 cm diameter stone found in the feces (37). When the stone is too big or when complications such as infection set in, an operation may still be necessary. Since surgery cannot remove minute stones which may be present, medication is still advisable after the operation.

4. Treatment of heart diseases

Although in China heart diseases are still treated mainly by Western methods (74), the author has learned through personal contact that in recent years many herbal drugs have been developed and used for the treatment of these diseases. One of the most important is Mao-tung-ching, developed in Canton. Also, a combination of herbs, the so-called "coronary mixture" has been formulated in Peking; and the combined Dan-seng injection for coronary diseases has been developed in Shanghai. The "Pin-liang-hua" extract, developed in An-san, Manchuria is used for rheumatic heart diseases.

4.1 Mao-tung-ching

There are three kinds of tung-ching, widely used in medicine and all belonging to the same family (70). They are:

"Mao-tung-ching (Mao-pe-sho)" *Ilex pubescens Hook et Arn.*
"Tung-ching (Shih-chi-ching)" *Ilex chinensis Sims.*
"Ti-tung-ching (Giu-pi-yin)" *Ilex rotunda Thunb.*

All three plants are grown in the southern parts of China. The root of Mao-tung-ching, found to be able to dilate blood vessels, is used in coronary heart disease. It can increase the blood flow in the coronary artery and reduce the blood pressure. Shih-chi-ching is used for burns (see below) and Ti-tung-ching is used for upper respiratory infections and gastrointestinal disturbances.

From October, 1970 through the beginning of 1972, the Chung-shan Hospital in Canton treated 103 cases of coronary heart disease with Mao-tung-ching (20). The treatment consisted of one course of 1 month or more, and the analysis of the results is as follows:

All cases selected showed clinical symptoms of coronary heart disease with abnormal electrocardiogram. Among the patients, 10 cases of acute myocardial infarction were also included.

A daily dose of 4 oz. of Mao-tung-ching was given to each patient orally. Most received supplemental muscular injections twice daily, each providing 20 mg of an extract of the drug (equivalent to 8 g of raw material).

It was found that 101 cases out of 103 showed significant improvement with a total effectiveness of 98.1 percent. Before the treatment, 98 cases suffered agonizing precardial pain. After treatment in 95 of the 98 cases the pain disappeared completely or was reduced significantly, giving a 96.9 percent effectiveness. All cases showed varying degrees of improvement in their heart function after treatment, and in 22 out of 38 cases of hypertension the blood pressure returned to normal or was lowered significantly

(57.9 percent). In around 70 percent of the cases, signs of numbness in limbs, headaches and dizziness disappeared after treatment. There were 60 cases with high blood cholesterol level at the beginning of treatment. In 30 of these the cholesterol returned to normal or was markedly lowered after treatment (50 percent). Among 89 cases with abnormal electrocardiogram, 32 cases returned to normal or were much improved (36 percent) and 53 cases showed no change (59.5 percent).

No marked effect was found on the blood picture or regular urine analysis. Although among individual cases there was a slight prolongation of blood clotting time after treatment, no bleeding tendency was observed clinically.

The largest majority of cases of coronary disease treated with this drug for approximately 1 month showed marked improvement. There were a few cases of recurrence but all were less serious. Toxicity was not found through the period (1 month) of treatment.

As shown by pharmacological studies, the active component in Mao-tung-ching has the following functions:

(i) It exerts direct action on the smooth muscles surrounding the blood vessels, dilates the vessels and lowers the blood pressure.

(ii) It dilates the coronary artery, increasing blood flow and nutrition in the cardiac muscles.

(iii) It lowers the cardiac muscular oxygen consumption.

4.2 "Coronary mixtures"

The author learned a great deal about the development of the "coronary tablet" for treating coronary heart diseases while visiting the Institute for Cardiovascular Diseases, Chinese Academy of Medical Sciences, Peking, through the courtesy of the director, Dr. Wu Ying-K'ai and his staff. (Although to date, their work has not been published, the author feels it is especially interesting and deserves mention.) It was found that two herbs, "Chuan-chiung" (*Ligusticum wallichii Franch.*) (Figure 21) and "Hung-hua" (*Carthamus tinctorius L.*) (Figure 9) when combined have a definite therapeutic effect on coronary diseases. According to the theory of Chinese traditional medicine, patients suffering from the same disease do not necessarily react in the same way to the same treatment. The individuality of the patient's physiological as well as mental condition must be taken into consideration and treatment must be given accordingly. With this consideration in mind, two types of prescription were prepared: One, designated as coronary mixture minor No. 2, contains only the two herbs mentioned above; the other contains additional herbs such as "Dan-seng" (Salvia miltiorrhiza Bge.) (Figure 36), "Chiang-hsiang" (Acronychia S. pedunculata (L.) Mig.) (Figure 3), etc. The extract from such mixtures is purified and can be given intramuscularly or intravenously, and tablets are also available for oral administration. In 1971, more than 200 patients were treated with these prescriptions with very encouraging results. Detailed information is expected to be published in the near future.

4.3 Combined Dan-seng injection

In Shanghai, another medical center of China, a processed combined "Dan-seng extract" is prepared (22) by extracting equal amounts of Dan-seng and Chiang-hsiang (1 g of each of these two drugs is extracted into 1 ml of fluid for injection). Dan-seng (Salvia miltiorrhiza Bge.) is the root of the plant. Chiang-hsiang is the center part of the root of a legume plant "Chiang-hsiang-teng" (Dalbergia odorifera T. Che).* This processed medicine has been found effective in dilating the blood vessels, thus increasing blood flow in the coronary artery. It has also proved useful in the treatment of precardial pain and myocardial infarction. Several hospitals in Shanghai have carried out clinical studies with this medicine in a total of 107 cases of coronary arteriosclerotic heart disease with varying degrees of angina pectoris. The method of administration varied according to the individual case; some were given intramuscular injection, others intravenous injection (1 ml of combined fluid extract diluted with 20 ml of 50 percent glucose solution); or intravenous infusion (4-10 ml of medicine mixed into 100-500 ml glucose or other type of intravenous infusion solution. Two to 4 weeks are regarded as one treatment course. Effectiveness is judged by the evaluation standard established in March, 1972 during the Chinese Conference On Preventive Medicine for Pulmonary Cardiac Diseases, Coronary Heart Diseases and Hypertension (22).

Symptomatic improvement results were: "Significantly improved," 24.6 percent (33/134); "improved," 58.2 percent (78/134); "no effect," 16.4 percent (22/134); "worsening," 0.8 percent (1/134). Electrocardiographic improvement results were: "Improved significantly," 18.7 percent (20/107); "improved," 29.9 percent (32/107); "no effect," 48.6 percent (52/107); and "worsening," 2.8 percent (3/107).

During the trial period, various tests such as liver and kidney function tests were carried out in some cases, as well as general blood picture studies and similar. Only a few patients complained of local muscle soreness due to injections. No side effects were observed.

---

*This scientific name given in Ref. (22) differs from the name given in Figure 3. However, the name in Chinese is identical.

From the results obtained through preliminary pharmacological tests, it was shown that the medicine has a remarkable tranquilizing effect on mice; it prolonged the effectiveness of hexobarbital without upsetting the natural harmony of sleep. An experiment with a heart perfusion (in vitro) found the medicine to be significantly effective in dilating the coronary artery and thereby increasing the blood flow in the artery when heart efficiency was already impaired. When the medicine was administered for the purpose of increasing the coronary artery blood flow, the drugs also improved the heart contraction, slowed down the heart beat, and thereby improved the heart efficiency. Furthermore, when this medicine was used to anesthetize cats and rabbits in experiments, it also lowered the blood pressure. When tested with mice by peritoneal injection, the medicine showed an acute toxicity as follows: $L = 61.5 \pm 5.26$ g/kg (calculation based on the Dan-seng content alone).

4.4 Ginseng and hypotension

Panax ginseng C.A. Meyer is a well-known cardiac tonic and is widely used in China (46). The Hua-san Hospital in Shanghai reported 7 cases of acute myocardial infarction with shock or cardiac arrhythmia treated with a combination of traditional and Western medicine (66). In these cases there was shock or very low blood pressure; the patients were extremely weak, with white faces, cold skin, cold limbs, sweating and very weak pulses; they were not alert mentally. When a Western type of drug was given to raise blood pressure, it rose temporarily but fell in a short time, even after repeated doses. When ginseng was given either alone or in prescriptions such as seng fu tang (ginseng, 15.60 g and cooked fu-tze (Aconitum carmichaeli Debx.), 12.48 g) (41), the blood pressure rose and remained at a normal level without falling.

Ginseng also is used to prevent shock, as illustrated in the following case: A patient suffering from acute myocardial infarction showed a tendency to develop shock as indicated by low blood pressure, white face and cold limbs. He was given ginseng, and 2 hours after the medication, his blood pressure had risen more than 20 mm Hg, his face looked normal and his limbs were warm (41).

4.5 Pin-liang-hua

Pin-liang-hua (1) (Adonis amurensis Regel et Radde) (Figure 4). This herb is widely grown in the snow mountains in the three northeastern provinces of China: Liaoning, Heilungkiang and Kirin. A local medical clinic at An-san found that it has a therapeutic effect on rheumatic heart diseases, particularly for those resistant to digitalis (1). Water extract tincture and powder were prepared and a number of chemical compounds, such as cymarin, adonin, adonitoxin, were isolated. These herbal preparations act as heart stimulants, strengthening contraction of the heart muscles and possibly dilating the coronary artery. A series of 32 cases of varying forms of rheumatic heart diseases were treated with the extracts of this herb at the An-san clinic. The ages of the patients varied from 16 to 51. The positive therapeutic effect was judged by the drop of the high pulse rate to 91 or below and by improvement of the symptoms and signs. Among the 32 cases treated, 11 or 34.4 percent showed positive effect in three days; 18 or 56.2 percent in 1 week and 3 or 9.4 percent showed no effect even 1 week after treatment began. The relative pulse rates are shown in Table 7. Among the 32 cases, all showed shortness of breath (22 of them improved), 28 showed liver enlargement and in nine of them the liver size was reduced; 29 showed various degrees of edema and in 14 of them the edema disappeared or was reduced. All improvements took place within 1 week after treatment.

Table 7

PULSE RATE PER MINUTE BEFORE AND AFTER TREATMENT (1)

Pulse rate pulse/min.	Below 76-90	91-100	101-110	111-120	121-130	141-150	161-180	Total
No. of cases before treatment	6	9	5	6	3	1	2	32
No. of cases after treatment	28	1	3	0	0	0	0	32

5. Treatment of burns.

The Chinese have in recent years made progress in the treatment of burns with herbal medicine. One of the traditional medicinal herbs, shih-chi-ching (*Ilex chinensis Sims*) (Figure 18), has been found very effective for this purpose (54). This herb is a cousin of Mao-tung-ching which, as mentioned previously (20), is used for treating coronary diseases. Recently, extracts of shih-chi-ching have been made and studied pharmacologically.

5.1 Pharmacology of shih-chi-ching

Shih-chi-ching has been widely used as an antiseptic agent (59). Each millilitre of its diluted solution, containing 0.0125 g of the raw medicine, is effective in the inhibition of *Salmonella typhosa*, *Shigella flexneri*, *Escherichia coli*, *Proteus vulgaris* and *Staphylococcus aureus*. It remains effective on the last mentioned organism even after a further dilution to each ml containing 0.00313 g of the raw medicine.

Pharmacological studies have been reported as follows (59): Preparation of shih-chi-ching was administered to rabbits orally or injected intramuscularly in experimental studies. The urine collected from these animals after 1 and 2 days following administration revealed that the drug retained its antiseptic function. This showed that this medicine is very stable even after being absorbed and metabolized.

Normal, healthy persons given large doses of shih-chi-ching (20 g powder, equivalent of 102.6 g raw material by oral route, or liquid extract equivalent to 20 g raw medicine by intravenous injection, or liquid extract equivalent to 40 g raw medicine by muscular injection) showed no signs of acute toxicity. Mice given lethal doses showed a series of signs of acute toxicity similar to lack of oxygen (rapid breath, convulsion and uncontrolled excretion).

By giving shih-chi-ching solution to mice, the LD_{50} determined was 233.2 $\pm$ 11.56 g raw medicine/kg of body weight. This is 194 times the adult human therapeutic dose (1.2 g raw medicine/kg). Thus the medicine has a rather low acute toxicity.

When rabbits were given a dose (10 g raw medicine/kg/day) 8.3 times the regular clinical dosage and continued for 2 weeks, their serum glutamic-pyruvic transaminase was 266.14 units, showing no significant difference ($P<0.05$) from the normal value of 257.22 units before the drug was given. However, the serum glutamic-pyruvic transaminase level was increased to 312.86 units 2 weeks after the rabbits were taken off the drug. This value was significantly higher than the normal level ($P<0.01$). It indicates that the liver function of these animals was somewhat affected. But the results of pathological examination showed only some mild infiltration of leucocytes, mainly lymphocytes, in the liver at the area near the artery. This finding showed that shih-chi-ching may be harmful to the liver tissue but only in a mild way.

After receiving the shih-chi-ching solution for a period of 2 weeks, the rabbits' blood NPN value was 34.8 percent. When compared with the normal value of 33.5 mg percent before the drug was given there was no significant difference. Two weeks after the drug treatment was stopped, the NPN was 30.9 mg percent, showing no significant difference in comparison with normal value. This result indicates that shih-chi-ching apparently has no effect on kidney function. Histologically, among the 14 rabbits receiving shih-chi-ching solution, 8 of them showed no inflammatory infiltration in kidney tissue; the other 6 showed a slight inflammatory reaction. This finding agrees with the results of kidney function tests.

Rabbits, in another experiment, were given shih-chi-ching extracts by intravenous injection. Various physiological as well as biochemical tests were then carried out. No significant difference was found between control and medicated groups after the rabbits had been treated for 1 week; neither was any found after the rabbits had been off the drug for 1 week. The pathological examinations showed a few cases of lymphocytic infiltration in some of the organs in both groups. This phenomena probably had nothing to do with the injections of shih-chi-ching.

5.2 Clinical results of shih-chi-ching

Although the herb shih-chi-ching shows very low toxicity after oral, intramuscular, or intravenous administration, it is used mainly by local application for the treatment of burns (54). The chief preparations for this purpose are shih-chi-ching (*Ilex chinensis Sims*) solution, and shih-chi-ching creams No. 1 and No. 2.

Since 1969 the Nantung Medical College, Nantung, has treated 225 cases of burns, mainly second and third-degree, with shih-chi-ching preparations. The patients were aged 2 months to 86 years. In 56 cases the burns covered less than 10 percent of the body surface; in 102 cases 10-30 percent; in 49 cases 31-50 percent; and in 18 cases 51-90 percent. Twenty-five patients, mostly babies and the aged, died, for a mortality rate of 11.1 percent.

In the treatment of second-degree burns, either painting or spraying with shih-chi-ching solution with exposure, or dressing with shih-chi-ching cream No. 1 followed by exposure, was applied. In the cases so treated, a brown or black crust rapidly formed. In superficial second-degree burns, the crust usually separated in 1 week or so, while in deep second-degree burns it sloughed off in 2-3 weeks with primary healing. In cases of early cracking of the crust resulting from pressure upon the wound surface, or infection under the crust resulting from septicemia, excision of the crust was carried out without delay and shih-chi-ching cream No. 2 with semi-exposure or wet compress followed by semi-exposure was applied. By means of this procedure, wounds were healed within 3 weeks. In early compound burns (deep second-degree burns complicated by third-degree burns), the wound surface was first covered with shih-chi-ching cream No. 1 dressings and subsequently left exposed. About 3 weeks after the burn occurred, debridement was performed, and the wound surfaces of second-degree burns were usually found to have healed. The granulating bed of third-degree burns was then grafted with small pieces of skin to cover the wound surfaces.

An ideal crust should satisfy the following requirements: Rapid formation of eschars, firm attachment, effective prevention of exudation and infection, permeability and capability of absorbing secretions, no increase of depth of the wound surface, and minimum toxicity. It also is well-known that an extensive, open wound surface can lead to loss of exudates, proteins, electrolytes and energy which leads to severe shock at the early stage, as well as to infection, causing incipient fatal septicemia. With shih-chi-ching solution and shih-chi-ching cream, preliminary observations have shown that both can form firm crusts with exudates from the wound surface, thus closing the wound and preventing further exudation by virtue of their antiseptic property and low toxicity. These clinical results have also been confirmed by pharmacologic studies.

Histologically, the crusts were composed of small powdered particles of *Ilex chinensis Sims* and fibrinogen.

The use of shih-chi-ching (*Ilex chinensis Sims*) in the early treatment of burn wounds presents two problems which necessitate further investigation and improvement of the medication. One is transient irritating pain (although this may be alleviated somewhat by four percent novocain spray), the other problem is the formation of brown or black crusts which can interfere with assessment of the wound depth and observation of the wound condition.

5.3 Shih-chi-ching used in an ointment for burns

At the Shanghai Second Medical College and the Shanghai Third Pharmaceutical Firm for Traditional Herbal Medicine there is prepared an ointment for burns (65), the chief ingredient of which is shih-chi-ching. The preparation is designated as ointment Yuchuang No. 10. Its preparation is similar to that of Western ointments.

Application of ointment Yuchuang No. 10 in the treatment of 23 cases of third-degree and mixed-degree burns was reported by the above-mentioned institutions, with special reference to its sloughing effect on eschars and to its local and systemic reactions. General information about the cases is shown in Table 8.

Among the 23 cases, the ointment was applied to 3-8 percent of the body surface in 15 cases and to 10-26 percent in 8 cases. The wounds in most cases were already infected.

In 14 cases in which the ointment was applied before the seventh postburn day, dead tissues sloughed off almost entirely, usually on the third-twelfth postburn day (average 8 days) with the formation of granulations ready for skin grafting. The survival rate of grafts exceeded 98 percent. In the other 9 cases, the ointment was applied after the seventh postburn day, and the time required for ointment application before the wound was ready for skin grafting was even shorter (average 5 days).

Besides the action of lysis of the necrotic tissue, the drainage of pus was obvious. All cases had large quantities of pus from the wound surfaces yielding positive bacterial cultures, but none developed sepsis. On the contrary, preexisting local infiltration gradually receded. Body temperature was slightly increased in 9 cases, being generally 1°C higher than the level before the use of the ointment. No marked changes were observed in WBC and differential count in the 8 cases in which the drug was applied to over 10 percent of the body surface. While systemic reactions were not serious in this series of cases, general supportive therapy was enforced because of the profuse discharge of pus.

Thus, according to the Chinese clinicians who are experienced with other forms of treatment for burns, the ointment Yuchuang No. 10 in combination with skin grafting is valuable in hastening closure of the wound and in shortening the course of treatment.

5.4 Burns treated with other traditional herb medicine

Over a period of 3 years, 500 cases of burns have been treated in a medical clinic of the Chinese People's Liberation Army, mainly with traditional herb drugs other than those mentioned above (18). The results are analyzed below:

Of the series, 290 were males and 210 females. Patients ranged in age from 3 months to 73 years. Causes of burns: boiling water 56.4 percent; oil flame 31.4 percent; other factors 12.2 percent. Severity of burns: slight, involving less than 10 percent of the body surface - 419 cases; moderate, involving 11-30 percent of the body surface - 42 cases; severe, involving 31-50 percent of the body surface - 21 cases; very severe, involving over 51 percent of the body surface - 18 cases.

Results of treatment: All 500 cases were cured. The duration of treatment ranged from 4 to 19 days in cases of superficial second-degree burn, averaging 8.7 days; and from 10 to 30 days in cases of deep second-degree burn, averaging 18.7 days. Among 40 cases of third-degree burn, the time for wound healing was 32.2 days without skin graft in 15 cases with burns covering 0.5-7 percent of body surface, and 44.8 days with skin graft in the remaining 25 cases with burns covering 10-84 percent of body surface. Wound infection occurred in 18 of the 500 cases (3.6 percent) but was cured by appropriate treatment.

The drugs used in the treatment of this series of cases were Burn No. 1, Burn No. 2 and Burn No. 3. Their preparation is as follows:

Burn drug No. 1: *Zizyphus vulgaris cortex* powder is mixed with 80 percent alcohol in the ratio of 1:2. The mixture, closely sealed, is allowed to stand for 48 hours, then is put through a press, filtered and the liquid bottled for use.

TABLE 8
GENERAL INFORMATION ON 23 BURN CASES (65)

Case no.	Age	Total burn area %*	3rd degree burn area %*@	Dressing Area %*	Dressing days **	Days for Skin Graft ***
1	4	5	1	3	4	12
2	2	16	12	12	4	12
3	64	33	24	4	5	15
4	1.5	75	4	7.5	1	10
5	33	19		15	6	13
6	4	13	3.5	6	4	11
7	2	13	12	2.5	6	13
8	19	25	6	5	5	12
9	21	48.5	9.5	6	13	18
10	46	15	11	7	12	16
11	66	23	16.5	3	8	20
12	47	50.5	20.5	26	7	15
13	21	70	1.5	20	8	13
14	36	41	19	7	29	33
15	38	13	6	5	2	14
16	17	32	13	3	4	12
17	17	36	11	5	4	12
18	44	94	5	18	15	22
19	1	15	4.5	6	6	9
20	14	44	30	12	15	19
21	29	62	21	12	10	15
22	51	42	18	21	7	13
23	12	20	14.5	8	8	16

* % of body surface.
** Dressing started on days after burn.
*** Days after burn ready for skin grafting.
% Not including mixed degree burn.

Burn drug No. 2: This is composed of five parts endodermal powder of lang-yu-pi (Ulmus campestris) and two parts powder of huang-pai (Phellodendron chinensis). The method of preparation is the same as that for Burn drug No. 1.

Burn drug No. 3: Four parts suan-tsao-jen (Z. vulgaris cortex) powder, three parts huang-pai (Phellodendron chinensis) powder, three parts di-yu (Sanguisorba officinalis) powder and one part kan-tsao (Glycyrrhiza uralensis) powder. These materials are sifted separately with a sieve having 0.48 mm diameter holes, mixed thoroughly and then transferred to 20-50 g bottles to be sterilized under high pressure.

Wounds are carefully inspected and prepared before medication; surfaces infected or badly contaminated are first debrided with bromogeramin. In superficial second-degree burns, the cuticle is preserved as much as possible and any blisters drained. With deep second and third-degree burns, the cuticle is removed. Because the drugs cause irritation, the burn wounds, especially fresh ones, are first sprayed with a small amount of 1 percent xylocaine. Sedatives and analgesics are used early in the treatment of extensive burns when necessary.

Generally, Burn drug No. 1 is indicated for fresh burns. Burn drug No. 2 is used on infected burns, and Burn drug No. 3 is used for extensive or excessively exuding burns, followed by No. 1. Initially, spraying is done 3-5 times a day at intervals of 3-4 hours. After crust formation, the number of sprayings is usually reduced. When no exudation beneath the crust is observed, medication is discontinued for superficial second-degree burns 4-5 days after injury and for deep second-degree burns 13-15 days after injury. Sesame oil is applied to the surface of the crust twice a day to accelerate sloughing. In cases of third-degree burns, early spraying is applied to keep the wound dry. Debridement of eschars and grafting are done within 15 days after injury. The wound is exposed to air after medication. To prevent crust rupture and hemorrhage, motion of the joints in the early stage of treatment is avoided.

In treating burns, especially extensive and severe ones, the adoption of combined measures is mandatory, including prompt antishock therapy, appropriate replacement of fluid, early use of oral herb medicine, selective employment of antibiotics, and other supportive measures.

6. Cancer therapy.

At the present time, the chemotherapy of cancer in China still relies on Western type drugs (35,38), including those developed by the Chinese themselves (47). Although hundreds of traditional herbs or prescriptions have been used in China for various diseases since time immemorial, the question of whether any effective cancer cure has been discovered in China was discussed with Dr. Li Bin, deputy director of the Tumor Institute and Hospital, Chinese Academy of Medical Sciences, Peking, and her staff. They have carried out extensive surveys and investigations in this field and have examined countless "cancer cure" agents and/or prescriptions obtained from throughout the whole country. Dr. Li Bin claims that the most difficult problem is the diagnosis of cancer, for not all cases designated as "cancer" are actually of this disease.

The recorded "cancer cure" agents fall into two groups: Minerals and herbs. The mineral group (mostly Archimedean-type minerals) often contains mercury or arsenic and is therefore highly toxic. The herbal group can be subdivided into three categories according to effectiveness: Those showing questionable effectiveness (patients who received treatment with the herbs experienced a sense of well-being but no real physical improvement); those showing temporary effectiveness (patients showed temporary arrest of cancer growth); and ineffective (patients showing no effect from treatment). In the second of these categories, the temporary arrest of cancer growth did not occur in all patients suffering the same type of cancer.

Generally speaking, the use of traditional herbs to help in cancer therapy should still be regarded as a profitable field for research. When cancer patients were treated with Western anti-cancer drugs, the simultaneous administration of herbal medicine sometimes resulted in improvement of appetite and general condition. Although it is difficult to evaluate the results statistically, physicians in China are convinced that certain herbs do have beneficial effects on cancer patients. As mentioned in Part 1, one of the general therapeutic principles in Chinese traditional medicine is to build up the patient's resistance to fight the disease-causing agents or factors. In cases involving cancer therapy, it is necessary not only to increase the patient's resistance against the cancer cells but also to increase the tolerance for anticancer drugs. In many Chinese research institutions and hospitals, scientists are now experimenting to find out whether herbal medicine, together with acupuncture, can counteract the depressive action of some common anticancer drugs on leucocytes and immunity-producing systems.

APPENDIX

PHARMACOGNOSY OF INDIVIDUAL HERBS DISCUSSED IN THIS MONOGRAPH

NOTE: There are many ways of classifying the medical herbs. The simplest way is to present them alphabetically according to their scientific names. Most of the herbs which concern us in the present writing are listed here with a brief description of each.

Achyranthes Bidentata Bl. "Huai-niu-hsi" or "Sun-niu-hsi" (7,11,19,30,51)

This herb belongs to the Amaranthaceae family. In China it is mostly cultivated, but some grow wildly in woods. The root is 30-90 cm long, and after being processed to dryness it is used as medicine (Radix Achyranthes bidentata). It has no odor and tastes slightly sweet. Ca-oxalate crystal can be seen from the cross section, and in the water extraction there are 5 percent of saponin and small quantities of oleanolic acid and glucuronic acid. In addition there is 8 percent of ash, which is rich in K-salt

In clinical studies, it shows an effect of lowering the blood pressure temporarily; has a slight diuretic action; slows down peristalsis of the duodenum and causes strong uterine contraction when excess dosage is used. The alkaloid contained in this herb causes hemolysis of the blood and denaturizes the protein.

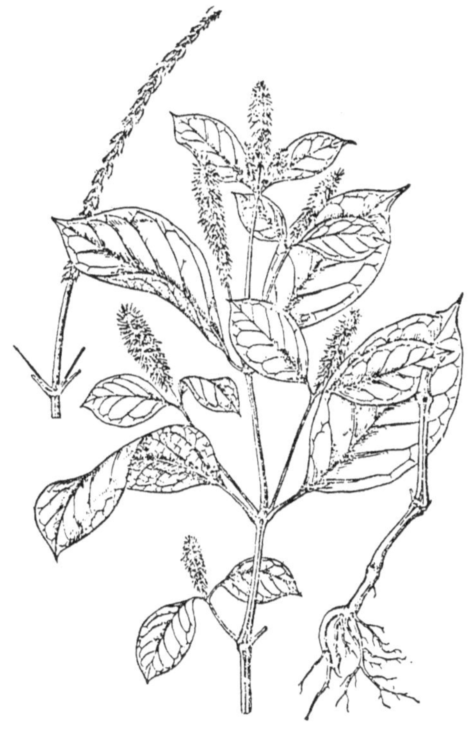

牛 膝

Fig. 1 Achyranthes bidentata Bl. (30)

Aconitum carmichaeli Debx. "Fu-tze" or "Wu-tou" (7,15,39,51)

This herb belongs to the Ranunculaceae family and grows to a height of 60-120 cm. The underground tuber roots, with four or five of them growing together, are used as medicine after special processing (Radix Aconiti Praeparata). Many of them have been cultivated in a large area in China recently. The herb's cross section has a characteristic layer called "Metaderm" which is a protective layer composed of epidermic cells. Starch deposit can be seen through the whole cross section. It contains 0.15 percent alkaloids, soluble in ether and about 30 percent sodium chloride. The alkaloids are mainly aconine and aconitine which are used as painkillers. The purpose of the special process used to turn this herb into medicine is to reduce the toxicity of the alkaloids.

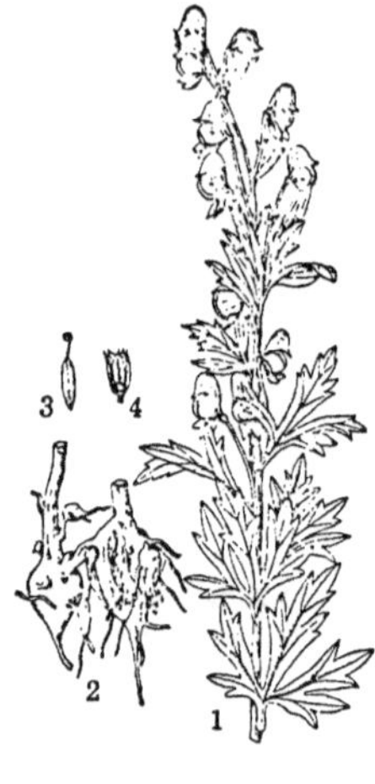

1. stalk with flower
2. roots
3. pollen
4. fruit

Fig. 2 Aconitum carmichaeli Debx. (51)

<u>Acronychia pedunculata (L.) Mig.</u> "Chiang-cheng-hsiang" or "Chiang-hsiang" (15,19, 23,36)

This, a small evergreen tree growing in the southern part of China belongs to the <u>Rutaceae</u> family. The center part of the stem is used as the medicine which has a nice aroma. Sometimes, the whole stem, as well as the fruit, are used as medicine. When the whole plant burns, the smoke generated gives out an aroma similar to that of burning incense. Preliminary chemical analysis gives the following results:

1. Under ultraviolet light: fluorescent spots at RF 0.13-0.22 fluorescent spots at Rf 0.25-0.49

2. Dragendorff's reagent test: no color change

3. Iodine (alcoholic solution) test: no color change

4. Platinic iodide test for alkaloid: no color change

5. Hemolytic test: positive (rf 0.4-0.84)

The main clinical application is to stop bleeding and pain. The pleasant aroma, which is probably generated from the plant's volatile oil, also provides a soothing effect.

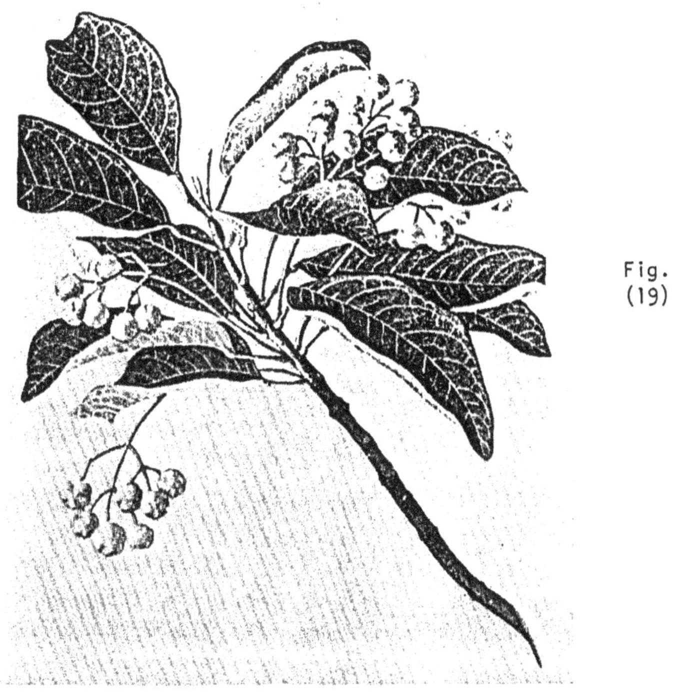

Fig. 3 (19)

Adonis amurensis Regel et Radde "Pin-liang-hua" or "Fu-she-tsao" (1,4,7,15)

A herb which belongs to the Ranunculaceae family; height about 10-40 cm. It is widely grown in cold regions (northern China as well as Korea and northern Japan). The whole plant is used as medicine (Herba Adonidis), has a bitter taste and is slightly toxic.

The main component is cymarin which can be hydrolyzed into cymarose and cymarigenin. It has a direct action on heart muscle, causes contraction, and also acts through control of the vagus nerves. It dilates coronary blood vessels to increase the blood flow. Other findings have shown that this plant also is effective as a diuretic and as a tranquilizing agent.

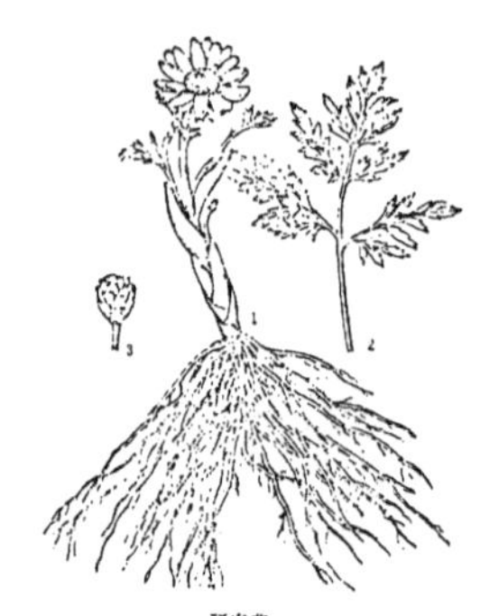

1. plant with flower
2. leaf
3. fruit

Fig. 4 Adonis amurensis Regel et Radde (1)

Alisma plantago-aquatica L. var. orientale Sam. "Che-hsi"(11,15, 19,29,51)

This herb belongs to the Alismataceae family; height, 50-100 cm. Grows widely in marshes in southern China. Its tuber stem with partial root attached is used as medicine, (Rhizoma Alismatis), and it has a slightly bitter taste but is not toxic. Sometimes the leaves and fruits also are used as medicine. It contains volatile oil, plant sterols, alkaloids, resin, protein, sugars, as well as fatty acids. In animal experiments, it showed some anti-bacterial action and it also seemed to lower the blood pressure, blood sugar and blood cholesterol. However, none of the components has been isolated to determine to which such action should be accredited.

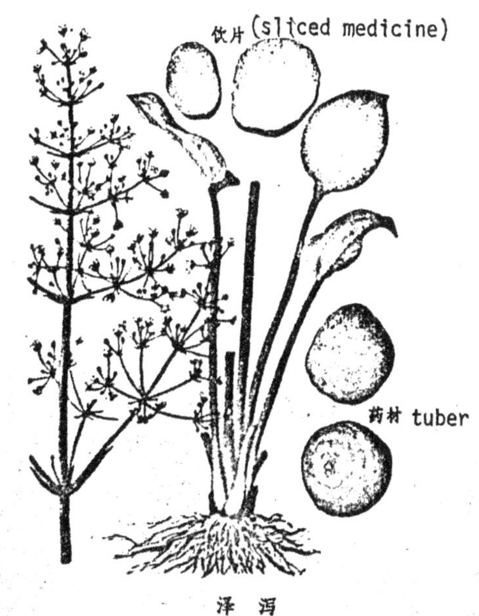

Fig. 5 Alisma plantago-aquatica L. var. orientale Sam. (11)

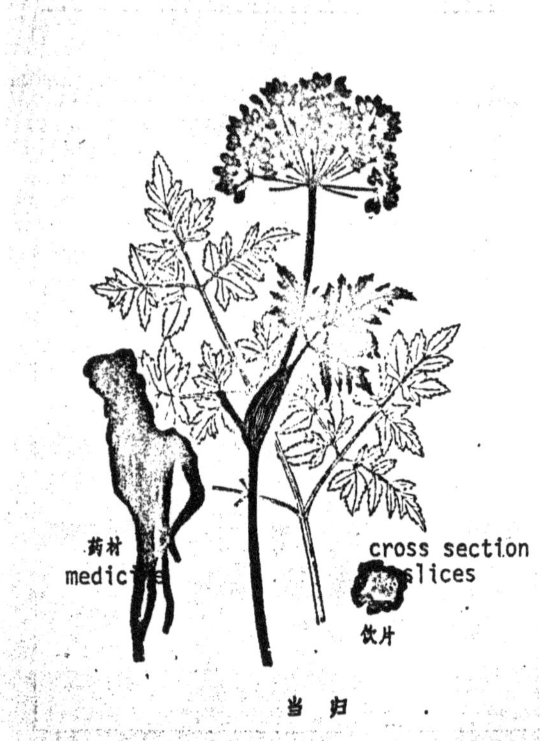

Fig. 6 *Angelica sinensis* (Oliv.) Diels (11)

Angelica sinensis (Oliv.) Diels "Tang-kuei" (4,11,19, 39,51)

This aromatic herb belongs to the Umbelliferae family, and grows to a height of 40-100 cm. Its main root is tuber-like and its branch roots are much longer. Both are used as medicine (Radix Angelica sinensis). The herb grows widely in high mountains and in plateau areas where it is cool and damp. The dried roots have a special aroma and a slightly sweet taste.

The special aroma mainly comes from its aromatic compounds such as n-butyliden-phthalide, n-valerophenone-o-carboxylic acid, n-butylphthalide-n-dodecanol and n-tetradecand, bergapten, etc. which are found in the roots. In the ethyl alcohol extract (3.4 percent), angelicone and angelic acid were isolated. Sucrose and vitamin E (77 mg/100g) were also found.

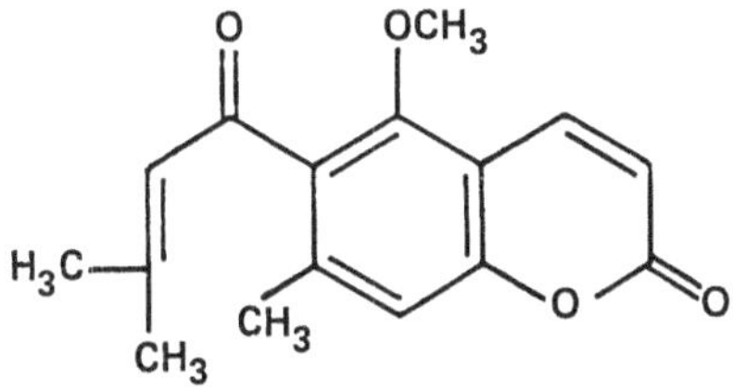

O OCH3 H3C CH3 CH3 O O

Angelicone

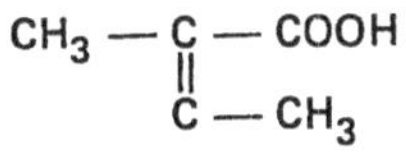

$CH_3 — C — COOH$
$\quad\quad\ \| $
$\quad\quad C — CH_3$

Angelic acid

The following conclusions were drawn from various experiments (39):

1. The injection of its water extract causes uterine contraction. However, when ethyl alcohol extract is injected, the uterine muscle relaxes.

2. It overcomes the symptoms induced by vitamin E deficiency.

3. It produces a tranquilizing effect on the cerebral nerves.

Benincasa hispida (Thunb.) Cogn. "Tung-kua" or "Tung-kua-jen" (15,30)

This herb belongs to the Cucurbitaceae family. It has herbaceous vines, and bears tendrils. The seed meal is used as medicine (Semen Benincasae); and sometimes the plant as a whole is used. In most of the oriental countries, this also is cultivated as a garden vegetable, because it has no toxicity. The main components in the seeds are urease, hispidamin, purine and trigonellin. It is commonly used for diuretic purposes and also in treating infant coughing. Mixed with other herbs, it is widely used as an external ointment.

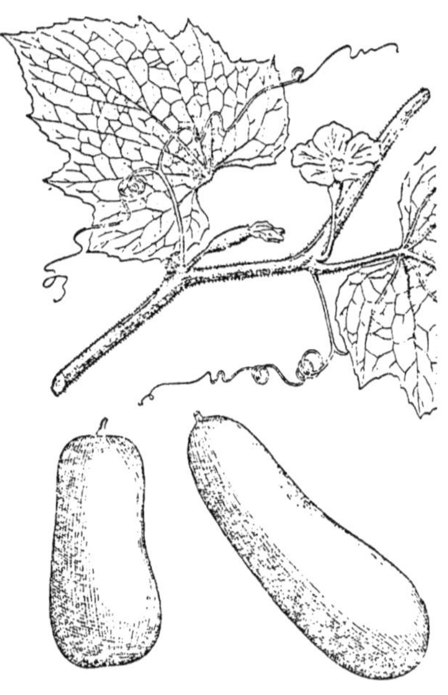

冬瓜

Fig. 7 Benincasa hispida (Thunb.) Cogn. (30)

Bupleurum chinense DC. "Chia-hu" (15,23,30,51)

This herb belongs to the Umbelliferae family and grows to a height of 40-70 cm. It is a plant widely grown in most of the dry roadsides and slope areas. The dried root is used as medicine (Radix Bupleuri) with a slightly bitter taste, but it contains no toxicity. The main chemical component is a-Spinasterol, $C_{29}H_{48}O \cdot 1/2\ H_2O$. In addition, there are also fatty oil, lignoceric acid and some volatile oil, etc. The important action of this herb is to reduce fever. Its extract is effective in treating malaria and other feverish diseases. The remaining parts of the plant, which contain rutin, also are used as medicine.

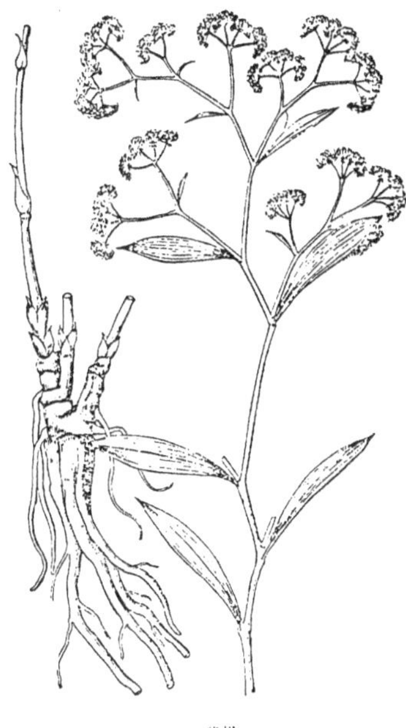

柴胡

Fig 8 Bupleurum chinense DC. (30)

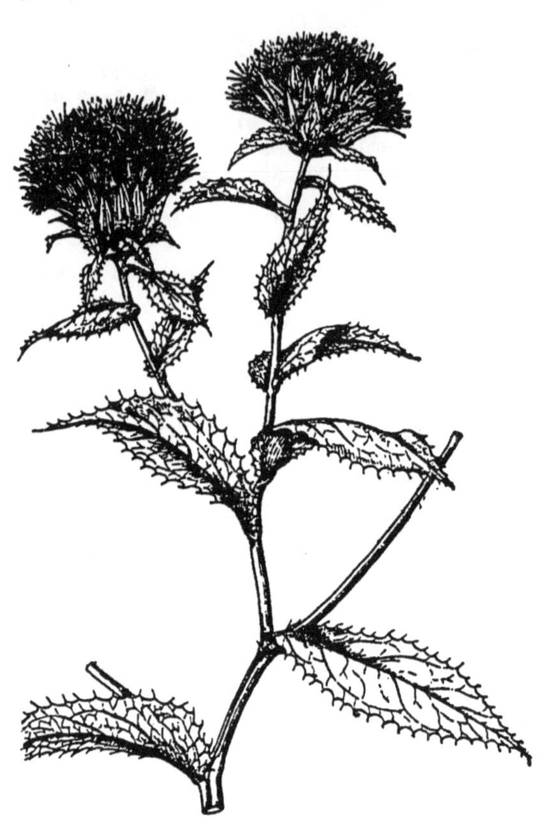

Fig. 9 Carthamus tinctorius L. (27)

<u>Carthamus tinctorius L.</u> "Hung-hua" (11,15,19,29,51)

This herb belongs to <u>Compositae</u> family, has a strong stem and grows to a height of 30-100 cm. The brownish red-flower at the top of the plant is used as medicine (<u>Flos Carthami</u>). It can be cultivated from seed in dry fertile sandy soil. The flower tastes slightly bitter, but contains no toxicity. It contains Carthamin (0.3-0.6 percent) and Safflor-yellow (20-30 percent) Carthamin is a red crystal with greenish fluorescence; it turns into Isocarthamin, which is a yellow crystal, after being treated with hydrochloric acid. When this compound is treated with 8 percent phosphoric acid, it can be hydrolized under CO_2 to become Carthamidin.

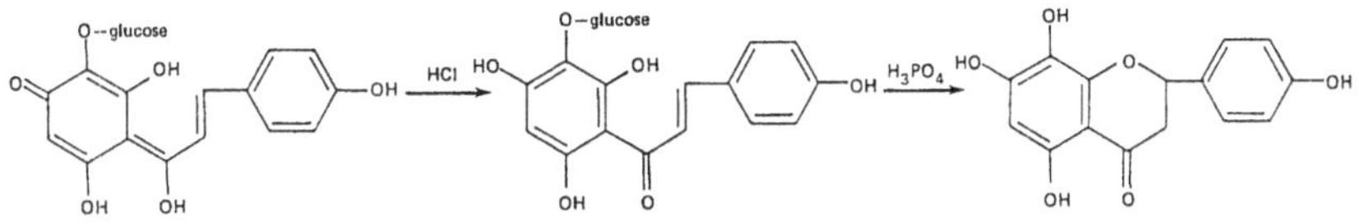

Carthamin —HCl→ Iso-carthamin —H_3PO_4→ Carthamidin

Externally, it is very effective in treating wounds to stop pain and in healing the wound. From animal experiments, it was found that this medicine has a stimulating effect on the uterus.

Citrus aurantium L. "Chi-kou" and "Chi-shih" (11,15,19,30,51)

The small evergreen tree or shrub is 4 to 6 m high. The fruits before ripening (Fructus aurantii immaturus) and after ripening (Fructus aurantii) are used as medicine. It can grow in most of China; thus it is widely cultivated. The skin part contains aurantiamanic acid and citval, etc. The mature fruit contains more aurantiamarin, a-limonen and hesperidin (a total of about 10 percent). Vitamin P is also present. It is generally used as an agent to help digestion and reduce gas pain.

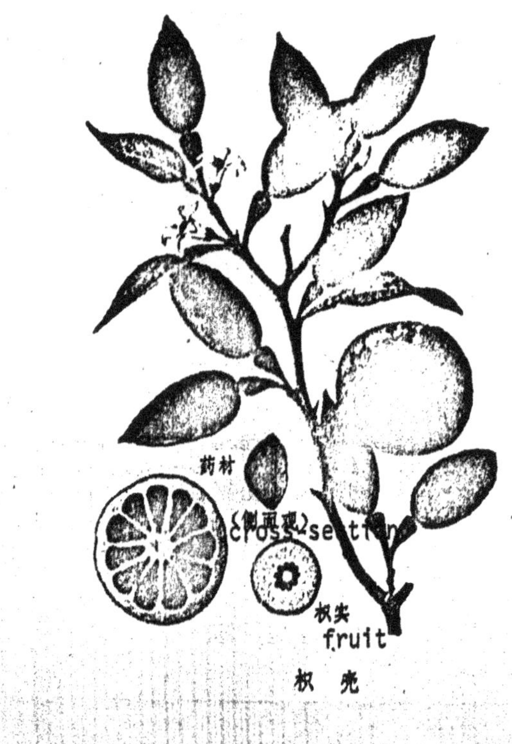

Fig. 10 Citrus aurantium L. (11)

Cornus officinalis Sieb. et Zucc. "Shan-chu-yu" (11,15,39,51)

This small tree belongs to the Cornaceae family and grows to height of 4 m or more. The dried fruit without the seeds is used as medicine (Fructus corni). It has an acid taste, and is slightly bitter and rather chewy. The chemical composition consists of cornin, gallic acid, malic acid, and other organic acids. Small amounts of vitamin A, saponin and tannin also are present. Traditionally, it is used mainly for general vitality restoration. However, in animal experiments, it has been found that this medicine has anti-Staphylococcus aureus and anti-Bacillus dysenteriae activity. In pharmacological tests, the diuretic and lowering blood pressure functions were rather significant. In the clinical studies, it was claimed to be effective in treating epidemic hepatitis.

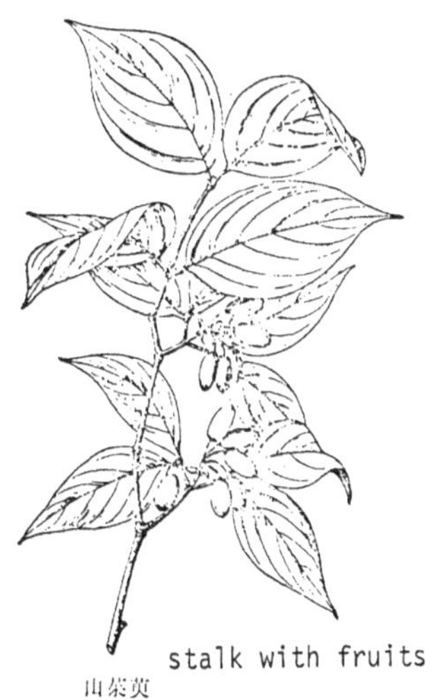

Fig. 11 Cornus officinalis Sieb. et Zucc. (11)

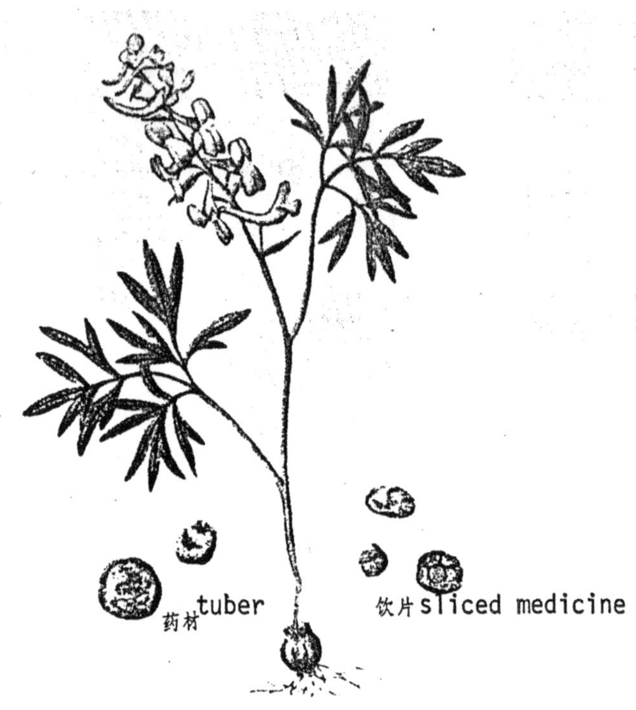

Fig. 12 Corydalis bulbosa DC. (11)

Corydalis bulbosa DC. "Yan-hu-so" (4,11,15,39,51)

This herb belongs to the Papaveraceae family and has a height of only 20 cm. The underground tuber stem is used as medicine (Rhizoma or Tuber Corydalis). It is very hard in texture and the cross section is golden yellow, with a waxy appearance which reflects a yellow fluorescence when placed under the ultra-violet light. It gives no odor and the taste is bitter. Studies of this herb found 13 alkaloids present. Some of them have been isolated as well as identified; these are corydaline, dl-tetra-hydro-palmatine, protopine, l-and dl-tetra-hydrocoptisine, l-corypalmine, corybulbine, b-homochelidonine, coptisine, and dehydrocorydaline. Traditionally, it was used to strengthen the circulation and to reduce pain. Pharmacological tests have proved that this herb or the alkaloids in this herb produce a tranquilizing effect which is useful in stopping pain or convulsion. At present, pills made with tetrahydropalmatine sulfate as a tranquilizer are already available for clinical use. The advantage of this drug is that it does not build up resistance, shows no habit-forming reaction, and its toxicity is negligible.

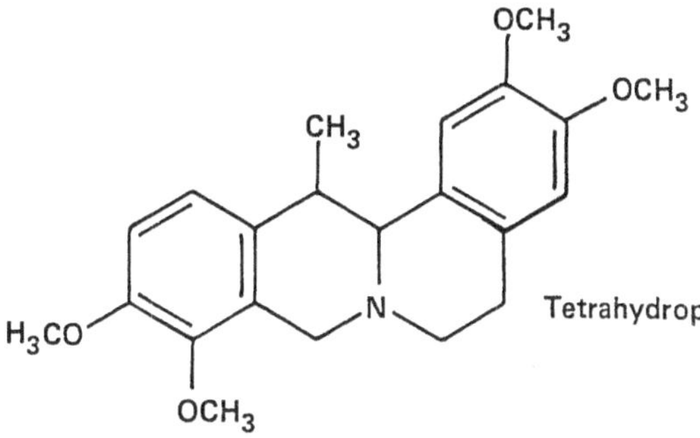

OCH_3 OCH_3 CH_3 H_3CO N OCH_3

Tetrahydropalmatine

Croton tiglium L. "Pa-tou" (7,11,15,39,51)

This evergreen tree, about 6 m high, belongs to the Euphorbiaceae family. The dried seeds (Semen tiglii) which are highly toxic are used as medicine. It contains about 40-60 percent fat with both saturated and unsaturated fatty acids, 18 percent protein, and 4-6 percent ash. The toxic element is the crotin, which is part of the protein component. In addition to the above, there are also small fractions of alkaloids, about 1-3.8 percent; the important one being crotonoside, which is similar to the alkaloid found in castor-oil seeds. The fraction in the oil portion which causes diarrhea is the croton resin (2-3 percent). This is a mixture of esters of phorbol with formic acid, butyric acid and tiglic acid.

$CH_3-CH=CH\cdot COOH$

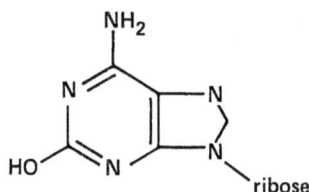

Crotonic acid

$$\begin{array}{l} CH_3-C-COOH \\ \qquad\ \ \| \\ CH_3-CH \end{array}$$

Tiglic acid

NH_2; N; N; N; N; HO; ribose

Cortonoside

Croton oil, extracted from the croton seeds can be used as a strong cathartic. However, it irritates the skin and mucous membranes, so the usage is limited. In recent years, it has been used mainly for treating schistosomiasis.

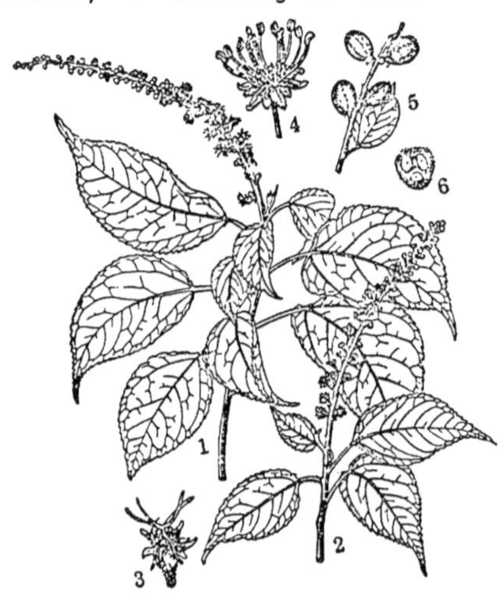

1. stalk bears ♀ flower
2. stalk bears ♂ flower
3. ♀ flower
4. ♂ flower
5. fruit
6. seed cross section

巴豆树

Curcuma aromatica Salisb. "Yu-chin" (7,23,39,51)

This herb belongs to the Zingiberaceae family and is about 1m high. The plant is cultivated mostly for medical purposes. Two parts of the plant are used as medicine: The tuber stem which is called Rhizoma Curcuma Longae (Chiang-huang) and the tuber which grows at the end of the roots, called Radix Curcumae (Yu-chin). This medicine has a slight aroma but no bitter taste. The main components in the volatile oil (6 percent) fraction are camphene, camphor, and curcumene with their derivatives. Traditionally, the herb is used for treating epileptic convulsions and circulatory disorders.

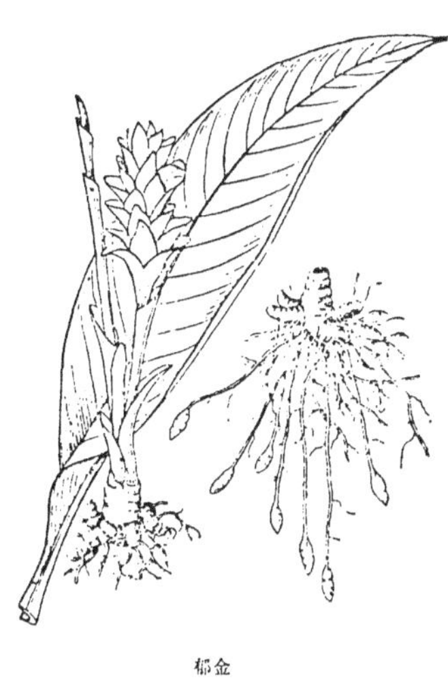

Fig. 14 Curcuma aromatica Salisb. (23)

Dioscorea batatas Dcne. "Shan-yao" (7,11,15,29,39)

This vine is a herb which belongs to the Dioscoreaceae family. The large tuber roots and the tubers growing above the ground are both edible. It is widely grown and can be cultivated in any area. The chemical composition is mainly starch with amylase, a small amount of saponin, allantoin, and mucin, etc. The dried powder has a soothing effect and is used as paste base for external application.

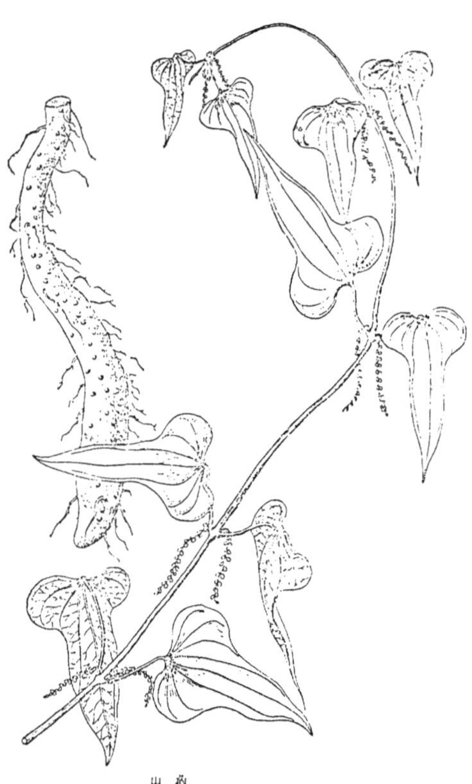

山 葯

Fig. 15 Dioscorea batatas Dcne. (29)

Euphorbia sieboldiana Morr. et Dcne. "Kan-sui" (7,11,15, 29,39)

This herb belongs to the Euphorbiaceae family and has a length of about 30 cm. The underground tuber root is used as medicine. The same variety of plants can be found in Japan. It is toxic, has a very strong odor, and a bitter taste. Its chemical composition consists of a- and r-euphorbol, euphadienol, palmitic acid, citric acid, oxalic acid, tannin, resin, glucose, sucrose, and starch, etc. Traditionally, the chief use is to treat edema. It is used also for constipation and as a diuretic. Externally, it is effective in treating local swelling.

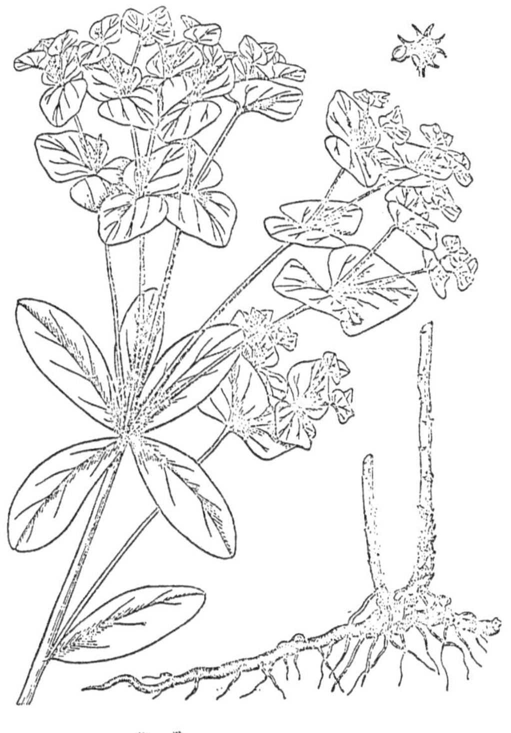

甘 遂

Fig. 16 Euphorbia sieboldiana Morr. et Dcne. (29)

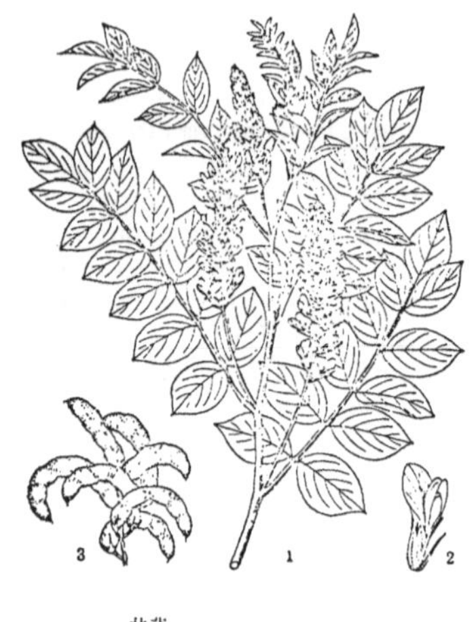

1. stalk with flowers
2. flower
3. fruits

Fig. 17a Glycyrrhiza uralensis Fisch.(51)

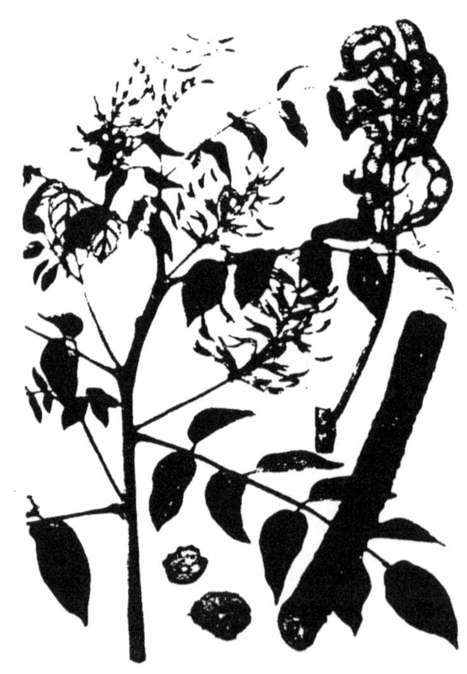

Fig. 17b Glycyrrhiza uralensis Fisch. (11)

Glycyrrhiza uralensis Fisch. "Kan-tsao" (4,11,39,51)

This is a Leguminosae family shrub with a height of 50-80 cm. It is widely grown in northern China and has been used as an important herbal medicine since the early history of China. The root and the lower portion of its stem are used as medicine after being properly dried (Radix Glycyrrhizae or Radix Liquiritiae). Its cross section clearly shows coarse fibrous layers with ray-like distributions. It has a very mild odor and a unique sweet taste. The chemical composition consists of glycyrrhizin (6-14 percent), glycyrramarin, liquiritin, iso-liquiritin, mannitol, glucose, sucrose and starch, etc. Glycyrrhizin is the compound that gives the sweetness which is 50 times sweeter than sucrose in the form of potassium or calcium salt of glycyrrhizic acid. It hydrolyzes into one molecule of glycyrrhetic acid and two molecules of glucose. Glycyrrhizin itself is a saponin and has no hemolytic action; however, glycyrrhetic acid will cause hemolysis. This medicine is widely used as a buffer in herbal compound prescriptions not only because of its sweet taste, but also because it serves as a filler for making pills. In pharmacological tests, it was found that this herb has a function similar to that of adrenocortical hormones. Clinically, it was claimed effective in treating stomach ulcer, duodenal ulcer and Addison's disease. It is also used in the food industry as a sweetener. Externally it has been used as an essential ingredient in ointments.

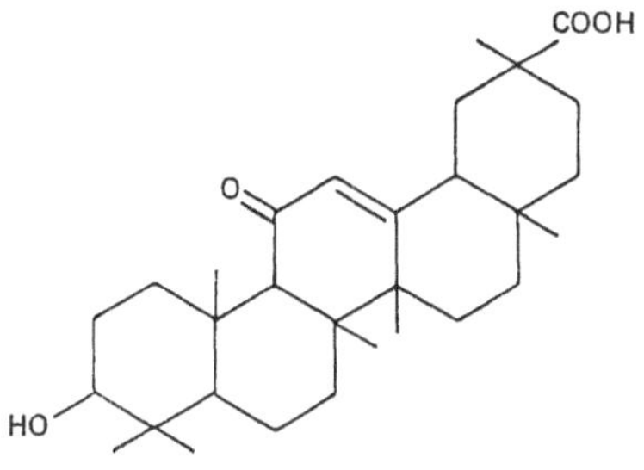

COOH
O
HO

Glycyrrhetic acid

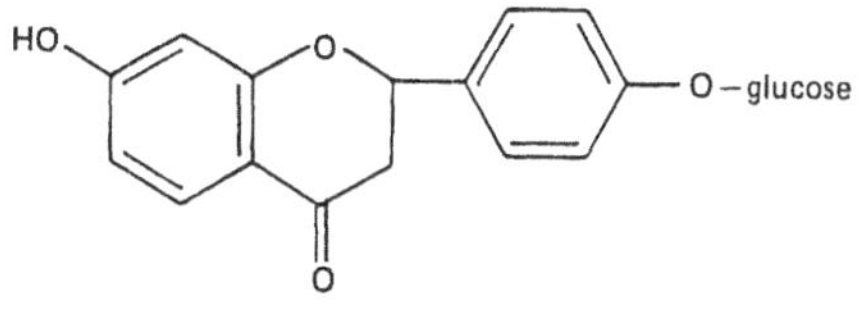

HO
O
O–glucose
O

Liquiritin

<u>Ilex chinensis Sims</u> "Shib-chi-ching" or "Tung-ching" (15,30,39)

This evergreen tree has a height about 12 m and belongs to the <u>Aquifoliaceae</u> family. Its seeds, bark, and leaves are all used as medicine. The bark contains tannin and some volatile oil; the leaves contain mainly volatile oil and flavonone. The detailed clinical application of this herbal medicine is discussed in Part II.

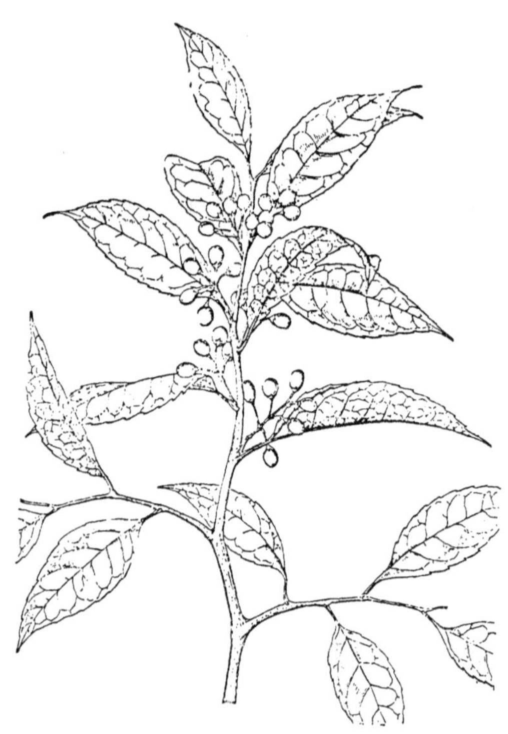

Fig. 18 <u>Ilex Chinensis Sims</u> (30)

Ilex pubescens Hook. et Arn. "Mao-tung-ching" (15,30,39)

This plant, either a shrub or a small tree with a height about 4 m belongs to the Aquifoliaceae family. It is widely grown in large areas as part of shrub woods. Both the root and leaves are used as medicine. It tastes slightly bitter but contains no toxicity. It is traditionally used for external application. More details are discussed in Part II.

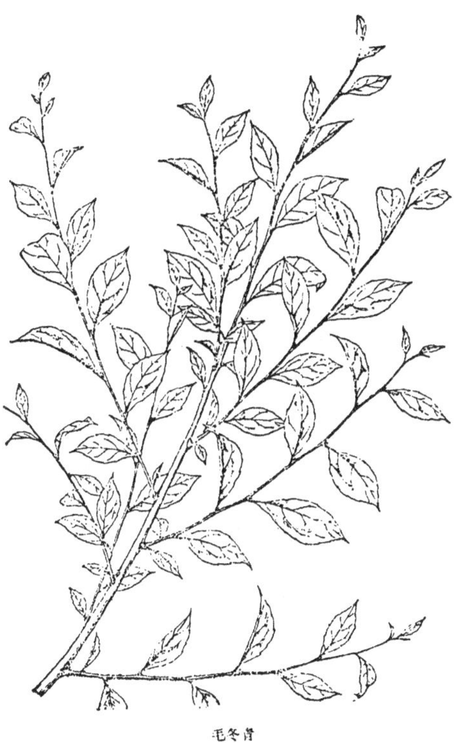

Fig. 19 Ilex pubescens Hook. et Arn. (30)

Ilex rotunda Thunb. "Ti-tung-ching" (19,39)

This is another variety of tung-ching belonging to the Aquifoliaceae family. It is an evergreen tree with a height about 10 m. The bark with its outer layer cleaned away is used as medicine. It tastes rather bitter (see Part II, Section 4.1).

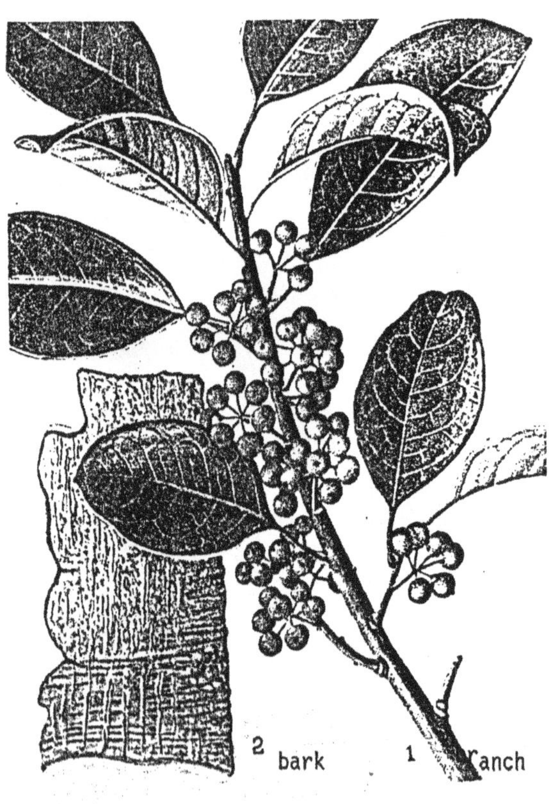

铁冬青（冬青科）
Fig. 20 Ilex rotunda Thunb. (19)

Ligusticum wallichii Franch. "Chuan-chiung" (11,15,39,51)

This herb has a height about 30-60 cm and belongs to the *Umbelliferae* family. It is extensively cultivated in China. The dried underground tuber stem is used as medicine (*Rhizoma Ligustici Wallichii*). Its cross section is yellowish and shows clearly the circular layers with oil spots. The oily-like alkaloid ($C_{27}H_{37}N_3$) has a peculiar aroma and is very bitter. In the volatile oil fraction, there is a kind of lactone derivative which is very similar to cnidium-lactone. In addition to the above-mentioned components, a small amount of ferulic acid (0.02 percent) is found.

Traditionally, it is used mainly for killing pain in cases of local swelling, sore, etc. Pharmacological tests have shown that the volatile oil extracted from this herb has a controlling effect on cerebral activity through the central nervous system. The drug made from this herb and now available in China is used to lower blood pressure, induce uterine contraction and also to stop bleeding after childbirth. In test-tube experiments it showed some antibacterial action.

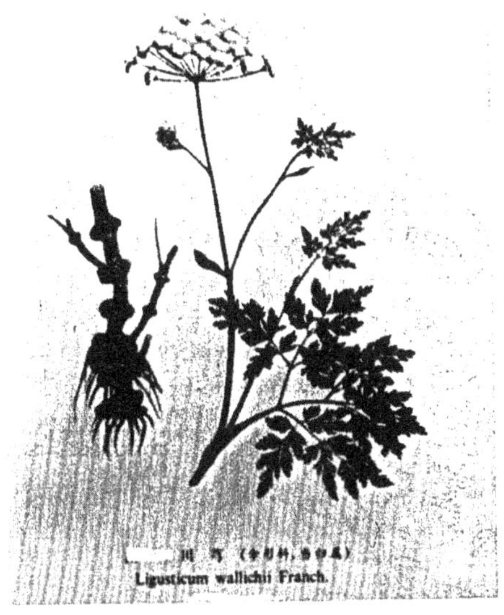

Fig 21 (27)

Lonicera japonica Thunb. "Chin-ning-hua" or "Shuang-hua" (4,11,30,51)

This semi-evergreen viny shrub is widely grown in all areas, and belongs to the Caprifoliaceae family. The flower is white when first in bloom, then turns to golden yellow after two to three days. Thus it derives the Chinese name, which means two colored flowers. The flowers are used as medicine (Flos lonicerae). It has a nice mild aroma and tastes slightly bitter. The important components are luteolin-7-glucoside, inositol, and saponin, the leaves contain lonicerin. Sometimes, the whole plant is processed and used as medicine. Since it has a general cooling effect, it is a rather popular drink among Chinese during summer. Experimental results show that it has an antibacterial action. It is claimed to be effective in treating influenza and other infectious diseases.

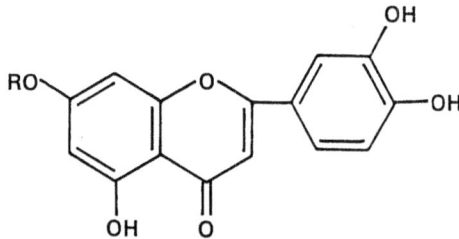

R = glucose for luteolin-7-glucose
R = glucose + rhamnose for lonicerin

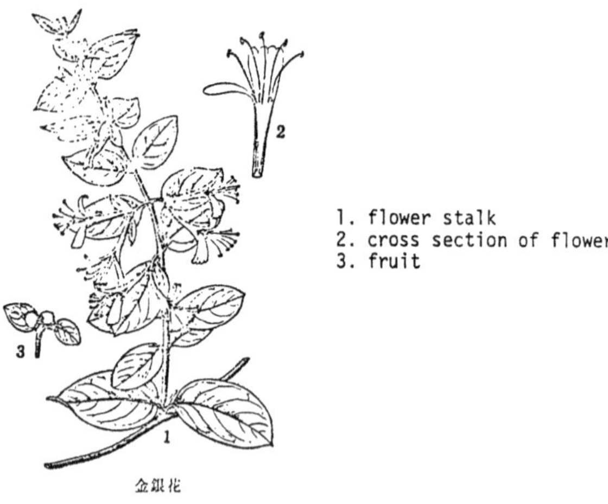

Fig. 22a Lonicera japonica Thunb. (51)

Lysimachia Christinae Hance "Chin-chien-tsao" (15,29,39)

This herb has climbing vines about 20-60 cm long with berry-like fruits. It is widely grown as roadside bushes. The whole plant is used as medicine. It has an acid taste, but is not toxic. It contains some phenols, sterols, quinones, amino acids, tannin, volatile oil, and choline. Traditionally, it is regarded as a detoxicating agent and is used in infections, inflammations, and wounds, as well as for all kinds of insect bites.

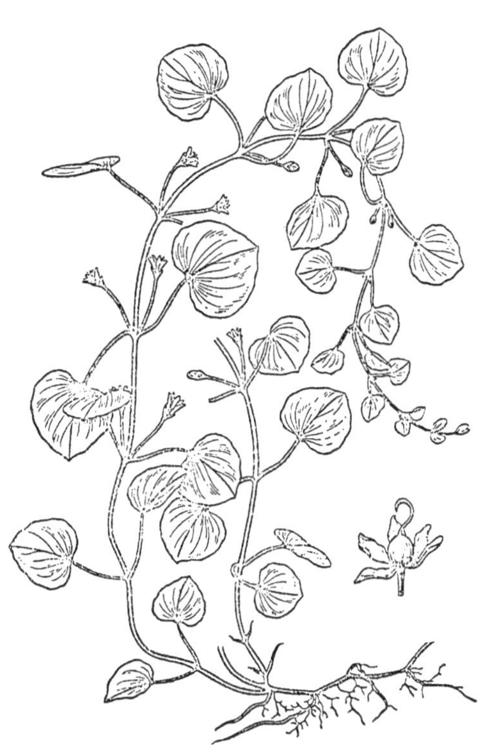

过路黄
Fig. 23 Lysimachia Christinae Hance (29)

Magnolia officinalis Rehd. et Wils. "Hou-pu" (11,15,29,51)

This tree, about 7-10 m tall, belongs to the Magnoliaceae family. The bark of the tree, when it is 20 to 30 years old, is used as medicine (Cortex magnoliae). It has a nice aroma and is slightly bitter. Chemical composition consists of 1 percent volatile oil in which b-eudesmol, magnolol (5 percent), and iso-magnolol are found. In addition, there are 0.07 percent alkaloids and about 0.45 percent saponin. Traditionally, the herb is used for respiratory congestion. However, experimental results showed that the extract has anti-Salmonella typhosa and other antibacterial actions.

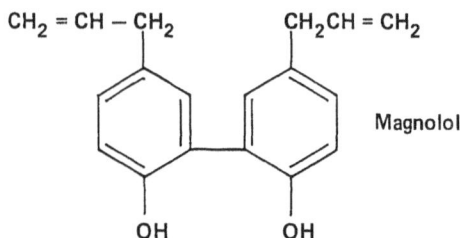

$CH_2 = CH - CH_2$ $\qquad$ $CH_2CH = CH_2$

OH $\qquad$ OH

Magnolol

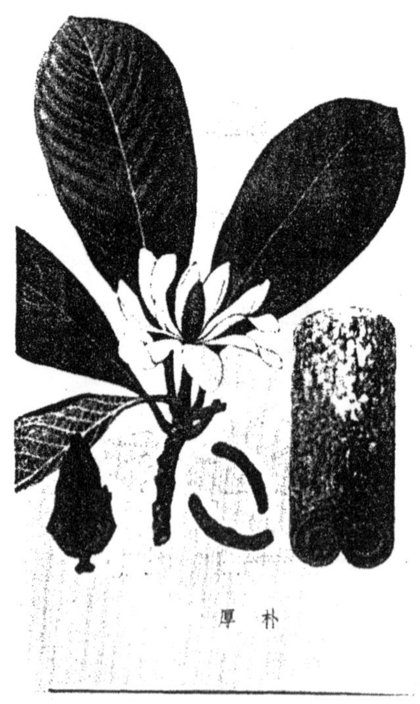

Fig. 24 Magnolia officinalis Rehd. et Wils. (11)

Melia toosendan Sieb. et Zucc. "Chuan-lien-pi" (11,39,51)

This tree with a height of 10 m or more belongs to the Meliaceae family. It grows widely in woody areas and the bark of its stem or root are used as medicine (Cortex meliae). It has no odor but tastes very bitter. The bitter taste component is the crystalline alkaloid, margosine. In addition, there are neutral resin and tannin present. The latter is the main component which is effective in treating parasites. There is also about 0.20 - 0.43 percent of toosendanin. It is also used as an ingredient in insecticides manufactured for agricultural purposes.

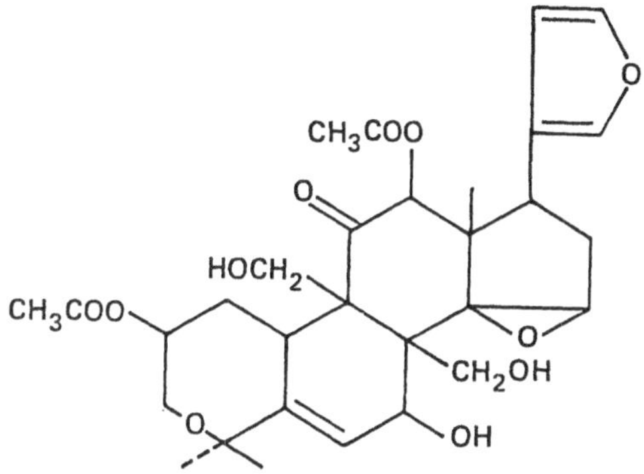

CH_3COO $HOCH_2$ CH_3COO CH_2OH OH

{178 ~ 80°
{233 ~ 40°

Toosendanin

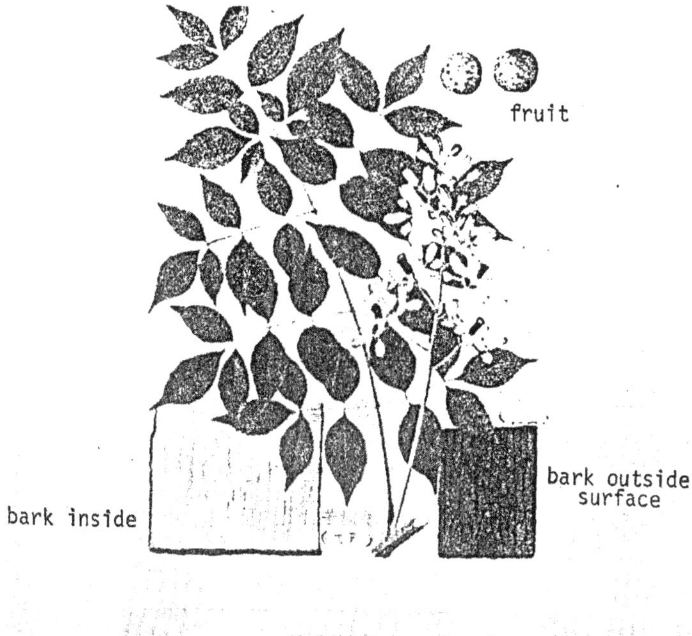

fruit

bark inside

bark outside surface

Fig. 25 Melia toosendan Sieb. et Zucc. (11)

Oldenlandia diffusa Roxb. "Pe-hua-she-shih-tsao" (15,30)

This herb is 20-30 cm long and grows everywhere as a weed in the family of Rubiaceae. The whole plant is used as medicine. Traditionally, the main use is treating heat stroke, however, it is also used as a diuretic agent as well as an anti-infection drug. Its chemical composition consists of a 31-C saturated hydrocarbon, stigmasterol, b-sitosterol, sitosterol-d-glucoside, p-hydroxy cinnamic acid and ursolic acid.

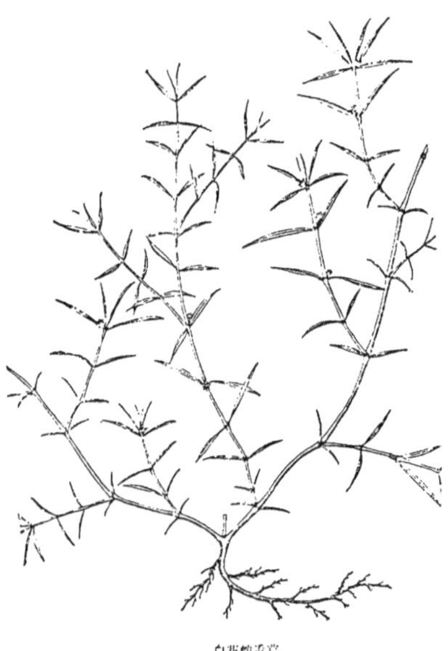

白花蛇舌草

Fig. 26 Oldenlandia diffusa Roxb. (30)

Paeonia lactiflora Pall "Pe-shou" (11,30,39,51)

This herb grows to a height about 50-80 cm and belongs to the Ranunculaceae family. The dried root is used as medicine (Radix paeoniae albae). When combined with a few other varieties of the same herb family the mixture is named Radix paeoniae rubrae "Chih-shou." All of these herbs grow wildly. However, there now are cultivated varieties in many areas of China. The root is cleaned free of its outside hard layer and small roots, before being processed as medicine. It has no odor and tastes slightly bitter. The chemical components are a small amount of volatile oil, benzoic acid, paeoniflorin, paeonol, and paeonine which is similar to aconitine. In addition, there are also traces of tannin, fatty oil, resin and starch, etc. Traditionally, it is used for improving general health. Experimental results showed that it has an inhibitory effect on pathogenic bacteria and on fungous infections of the skin.

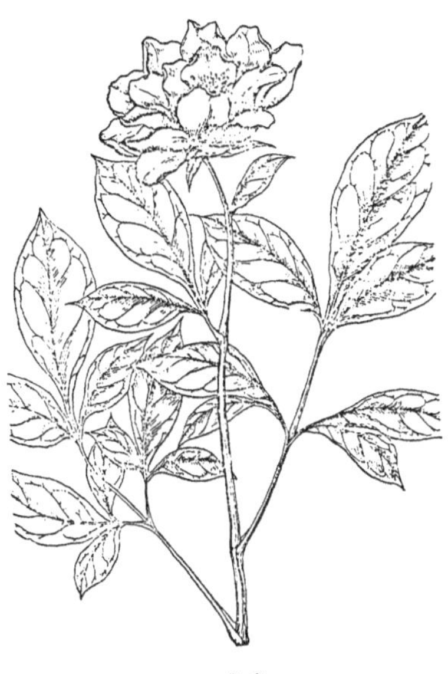

Fig. 27 Paeonia lactiflora Pall (30)

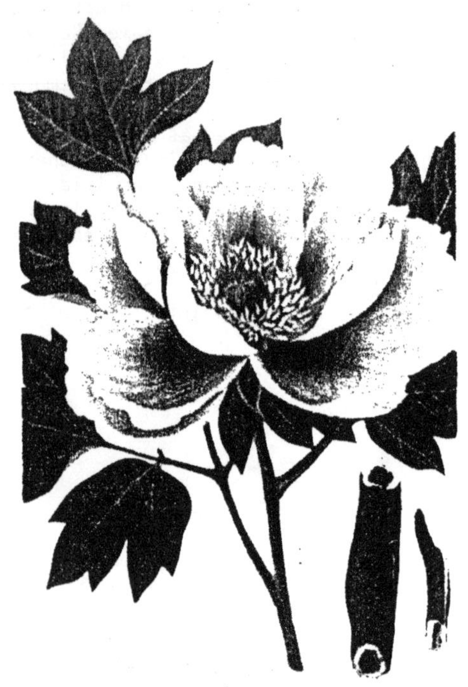

牡丹皮

Fig. 28 Paeonia suffruticosa Andr. (11)

Paeonia suffruticosa Andr. "Mau-dan-pi" (11,29,39,51)

This small shrub with a height about 1 - 1.5 m belongs to the *Ranunculaceae* family. The dried root bark with or without the outside layer is used as medicine (*Cortex moutan radicis*). It has a fragrant aroma and no taste. The cross section shows many deposits of starch granule and calcium oxalate crystals. Fresh bark contains paeonolide about 5-6 percent, which is easily hydrolyzed into paeonoside and paeonol by the enzymes in tissue. In addition, it contains 0.15-0.4 percent of volatile oil, benzoic acid, plant sterols, and about 0.4 percent of paeonine. Traditionally, it is used to reduce fever or to dissolve blood clots resulting from wounds. In experimental studies it was found that the herb has antibacterial and blood pressure lowering properties.

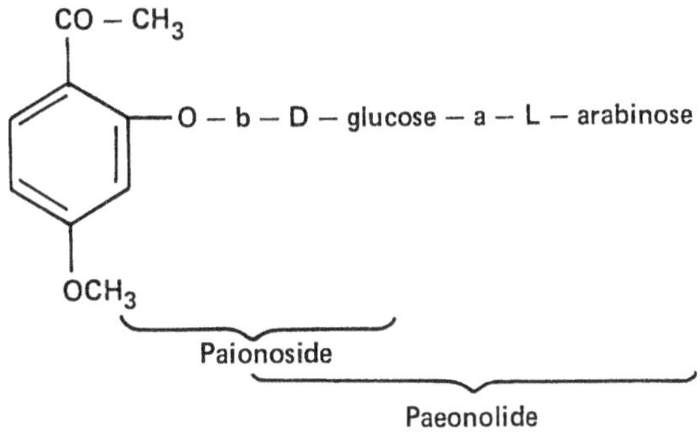

$CO - CH_3$

O – b – D – glucose – a – L – arabinose

OCH_3

Paionoside

Paeonolide

Panax ginseng C.A. Meyer "Jen-seng" (11,46,51)

This herb grows to about 60 cm in height and belongs to the Araliaceae family. The dried root is used as medicine (Radix ginseng). A detailed discussion of this herb can be found in Ref. (46).

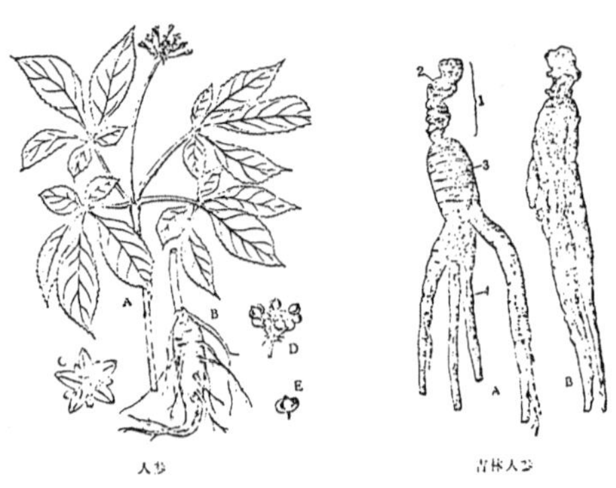

A & B are two varieties

Fig. 29 Panax ginseng C.A. Meyer (51)

A. stalk with flower
B. undergroung part of the plant
C. flower looking from the top
D.& E. fruits

1. whole head part of the root
2. bowl part of the head
3. main root portion
4. branch roots

Phellodendron chinense Schneid. "Huang-pai" or "Huang-pi-shou" (15,30,39,51)

This tree grows to a height of 10-12 m and belongs to the Rutaceae family. The dried tree bark is used as medicine (Cortex phellodendri). It usually grows in the woods. However, it also can be cultivated from seeds. The bark is harvested from the trees when they are 10 to 15 years old. The outside layer is scraped from the bark and not used for medicine. Its cross section has a bright yellow color and it has almost no odor but a bitter taste. It shows golden yellow fluorescence under ultraviolet light. The chemical composition consists of 1.4 - 4 percent berberine, which is also the main component, small amounts of palmatine, phellodendrine, and magnoflorine. In addition to these, there are also nitrogen-free compounds such as obakunone, obakulactone, dictamnolide, and some sticky substances composed of sterols and fatty acids. Traditionally, it is used to reduce fever in the treatment of dysentery and jaundice, etc. Recently, it was confirmed that this medicine is effective in treating dysentery.

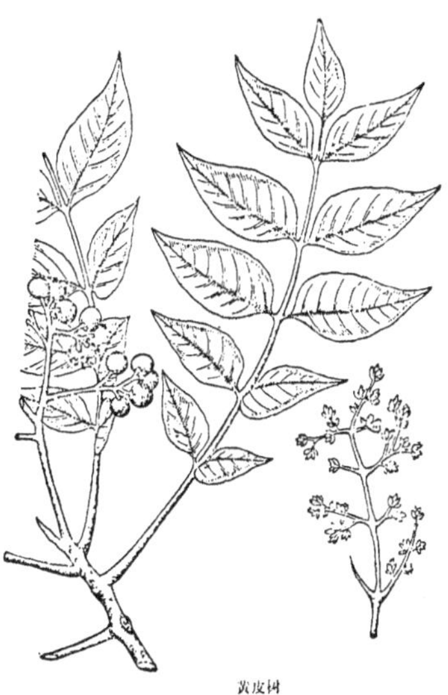

黄皮树

Fig. 30 Phellodendron chinense Schneid. (30)

Pinellia ternata (Thunb.) Breit. "Pan-hsia" (4,11,15,30,51)

This herb grows to 10-35 cm and belongs to the Araceae family. It can be found in most places where weeds are growing. The ball-shaped tuber stem is used as medicine (Rhizoma pinelliae). The cross section shows white powdery texture, with no detectable odor and with a little sticky taste. The cells are full of starch granules with various shapes. It contains b-sitosterol glucoside, choline and also small amounts of volatile oils, sterols, saponin, fatty acids, etc. besides starch. Traditionally, it is used to clear congestion in the respiratory system, to relieve gas pain and vomiting during pregnancy. Pharmacological tests confirmed its anti-vomiting action.

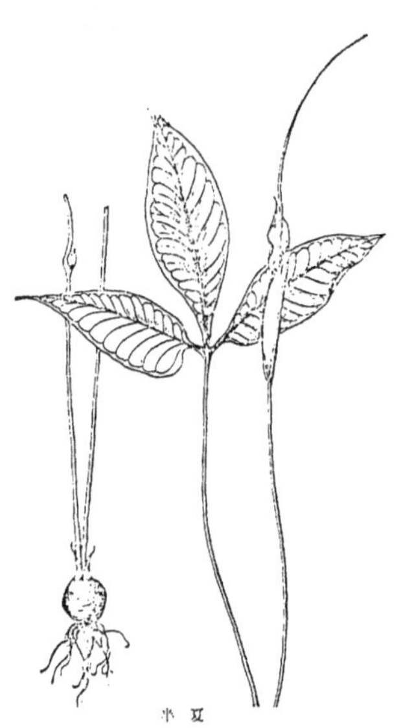

Fig. 31 Pinellia ternata (Thunb.) Breit (30)

Poria cocos (Schw.) Wolf. "Fu-lin" (11,15,39,51)

This is a parasitic growth, a kind of fungus that belongs to the Polyporaceae family. Mostly, it grows on the roots of old pine trees, about 20-30 cm. underground in various tuberous shapes. In recent years, cultivation has been very successful. It contains pachymic acid ($C_{33}H_{52}O_5$) and b-pachyman, a kind of polysaccharide which comprises 93 percent of the total components. Besides, there are small amounts of ergosterol, choline, phospholipids, proteins, resin, fats and enzymes, etc. Traditionally, it is used as a diuretic agent for treating edema, in soothing coughs and as a tranquilizing agent. Pharmacological testing proved the diurectic action, and also found that it can lower the blood sugar level. However, it did not show the tranquilizing effect.

HOOC

OH

CH_3COO

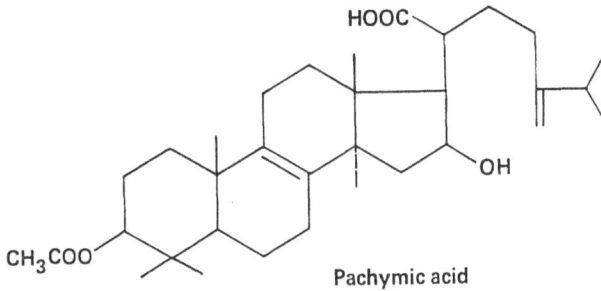

Pachymic acid

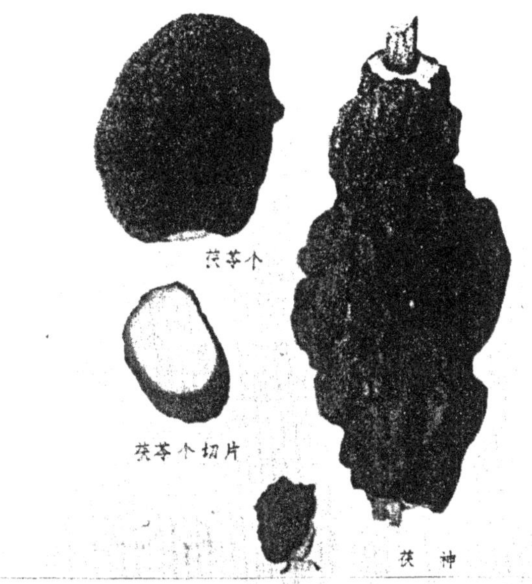

Fig. 32 Poria cocos (Schw.) Wolf (11)

Prunus persica (L.) Batsch "Tao-jen" (11,15,29,39,51)

This shrub or small tree belongs to the *Rosaceae* family. It grows to a height of 1-4 m. The dried ripe seeds are used as medicine (*Semen persicae*). It has no toxicity and tastes slightly bitter. The chemical composition consists of high levels of fatty oil and small amount of amygdalin.

CN
HC
O–glucose–glucose

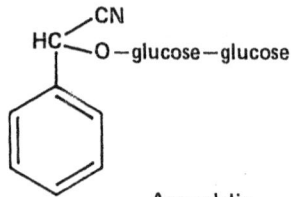

Amygdalin

Traditionally, it is used for general disturbances of the digestive tract. It is a mild helpful agent in constipation.

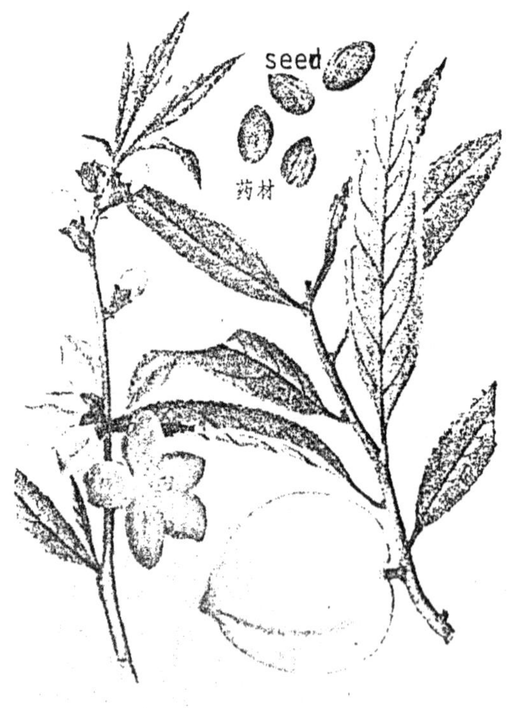

桃 仁

Fig. 33 *Prunus persica (L.) Batsch* (11)

Rehmannia glutinosa (G.) Libosch. "Di-huang" (11,15,29, 39,51)

This herb with a height about 10-40 cm belongs to the Scrophulariaceae family. The tuber root is used as a medicine (Radix rehmanniae). In recent years, this plant has been cultivated successfully; however, the wild supply is still plentiful. Its cross section is black and very dense in texture. It has almost no odor and a sweet taste. It contains mannitol and glucose in addition to the alcohol soluble rehmannin. Traditionally, it is used mainly to reduce fever in any illness. Pharmacological tests have found that this herb is effective as a stimulant for the heart, as a diuretic agent and in lowering blood sugar.

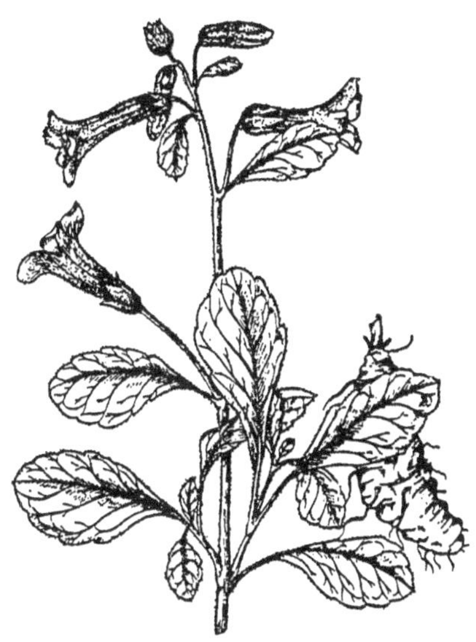

Fig. 34 Rehmannia glutinosa (G.) Libosch. (55)

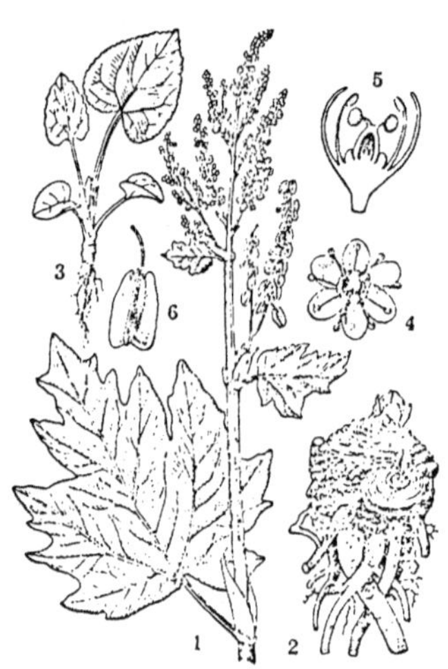

1. stalk with flower & fruit
2. root
3. seedling
4. flower looking from the top
5. flower cross section
6. fruit

Fig. 35 Rheum tanguticum Maxim. ex Rgl. (51)

Rheum tanguticum Maxim. et Rgl. "Ta-huang" (4,11,39,51)

This herb, which has been an export item to the European countries from China since 100 B.C., is really a specialty, and it presently is still exported. It grows to a height of about 2 m and belongs to the Polygonaceae family. The herb is a semicultivated plant growing on cold high land (2000-4000 m. above sea level). The dried root stem is used as medicine (Rhizoma rhei). Its cross section or its powder shows a brownish fluorescence under ultraviolet light. It has a unique aroma and a bitter taste. Its chemical composition consists of 2-5 percent of glucosides and quinone derivatives, in which the free quinone derivatives, such as rhein, emodin, chrysophanol, aloe-emodin and physcion are only about 1/10-1/5 of the total amount. In addition to these, there are about 5 percent tannins such as glucogallin, gallic acid and d-getechin, as well as small amounts of resin, dextrin, starch and sugars.

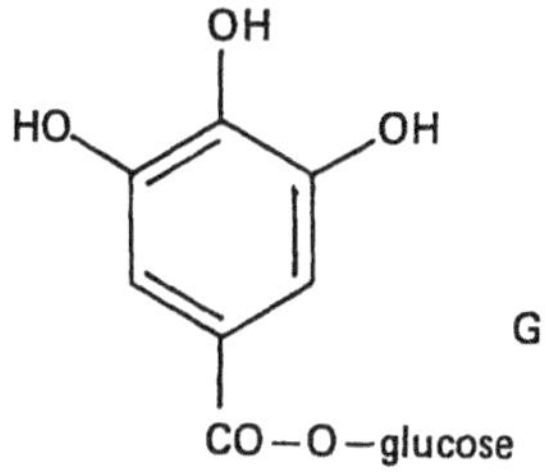

OH
HO OH
CO—O—glucose

Glucogallin

This herb is the most effective agent for non-habitual constipation. Its potency is directly proportional to the content of the conjugated form of rhein. The free form has no diarrhetic action. It is also used in industry as a yellow dye.

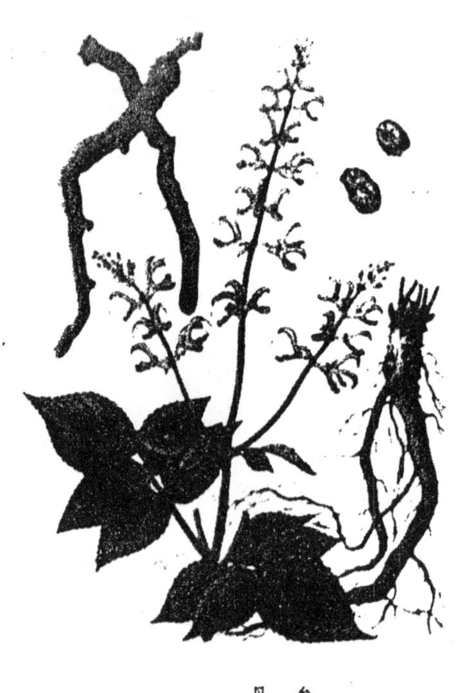

Fig. 36 Salvia miltiorrhiza Bge. (11)

Salvia miltiorrhiza Bge. "Dan-seng" (11,15,39,51)

This herb, with a height of about 20-80 cm, belongs to the Labiatae family. The dried root is used as medicine (Radix salviae miltiorrhizae). Most of the supply grows wildly; some is cultivated. The cross section is very fibrous with a ray-like arrangement. It has almost no odor, and is slightly bitter. The following components are already isolated and identified: Tanshinone I is a purplish-brown small sheet-like crystal; tanshinone II is a red small sheet-like crystal; and cryptotanshinone is an orange colored sheet-like crystal.

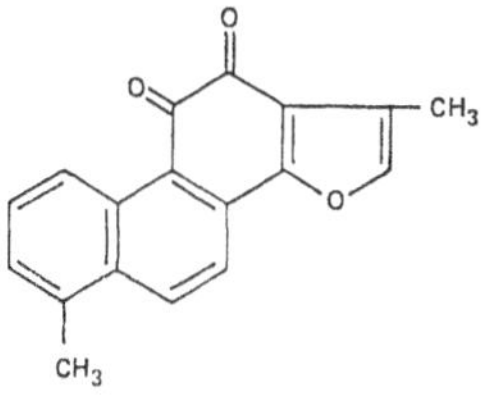

Tanshinone I

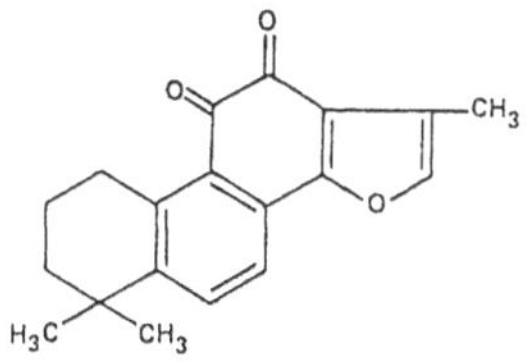

Tanshinone II

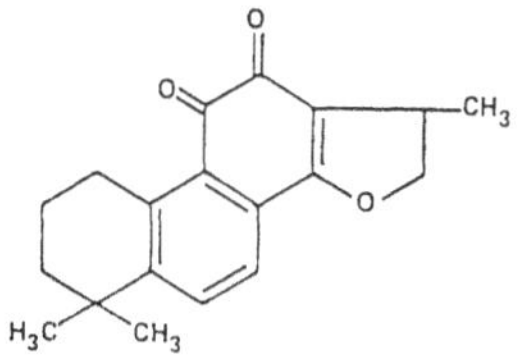

Cryptotanshinone

In addition to these, there are also tanshinol I, tanshinol II and vitamin E. Traditionally it is used for ailments related to circulation. It also was believed that the herb is effective in treating nervous insomnia, enlargement of the spleen and hypertension. However, experimental tests have shown that in the test tube, it has an inhibiting action on Bacillus pyocyaneus, Vibrio cholerae, and Bacillus dysenteriae. Moreover, it has a very strong inhibitory action on Staphylococcus aureus. It also showed some inhibition of dermatophytes.

Sanguisorba officinalis L. "Di-yu" (11,15,29,51)

This herb has a height of about 50-150 cm and belongs to the Rosaceae family. There are a few tuber roots at the end of a woody stem which is used as medicine (Radix sanguisorbae). The cross section is pinkish or light yellowish brown in color with fibrous bundles arranged in ray-like white spots. It has almost no odor, and a slightly bitter taste. It contains tannin, and sanguisorbin ($C_{38}H_{60}O_7$) which separates into sanguisorbigenin and valeric acid upon hydrolysis. Traditionally, it is used for stopping bleeding, particularly hemorrhage in dysentery, and vomiting and bleeding after childbirth. Externally, it can be used in burns, snakebite and insect bites.

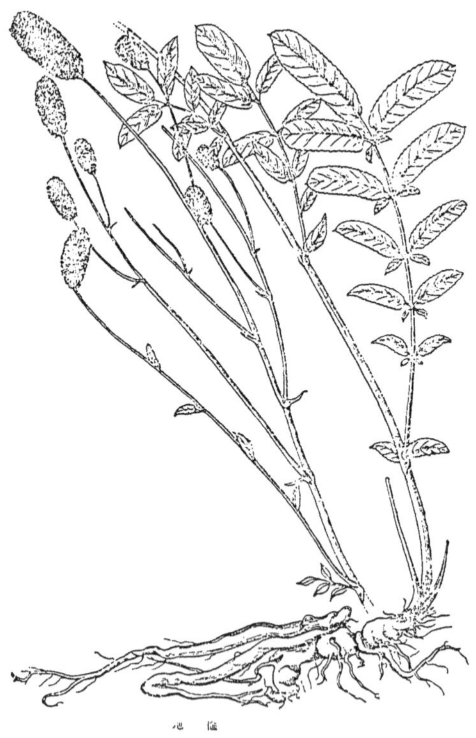

Fig. 37 Sanguisorba officinalis L. (29)

Sargentodoxa cuneata (Oliv.) Rehd. et Wils. "(Ta-hsueh-teng"
(11,29)

This tiny shrub grows to about 10 m and belongs to the Leguminosae family. The whole plant, free from leaves and small branches, is used as medicine. The plant can be found almost everywhere. It tastes bland; sometimes can be slightly bitter, but it has no toxicity. Traditionally, it is used against parasites, especially hookworm, and also is used to stop pain in amenorrhea and miscarriage cases.

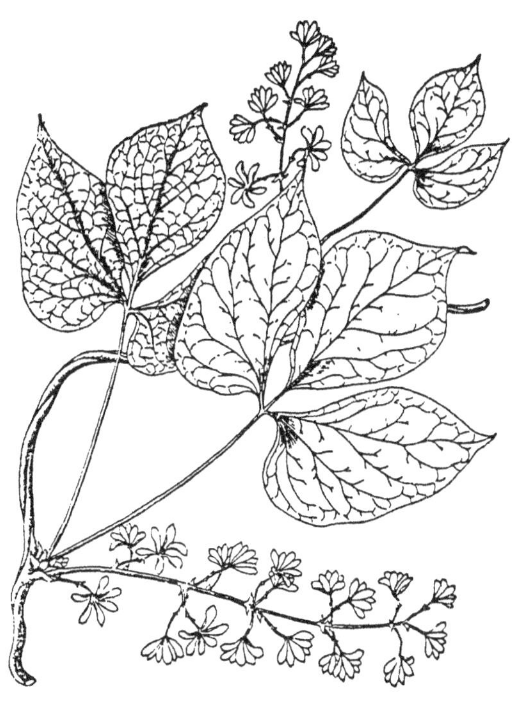

大血藤

Fig. 38 Sargentodoxa cuneata (Oliv.) Rehd. et Wils. (29)

Saussurea lappa Clarke "Mu-hsiang" (11,39,51)

This large herb, about 1-2 m high, belongs to the Compositae family. Originally, it was imported from India; however, it has been cultivated in many high altitude areas (2500-4000 m above sea level) of China in recent years. The dried roots are used as medicine (Radix saussureae lappae). The cross section is rather smooth, light yellow to dark brown with large brownish shiny oil chambers scattered around and easily seen. The aroma is very strong and unique, and it has taste. It contains 1-2.8 percent volatile oil, 6 percent resin, 0.05 percent saussurine, and about 18 percent sugars. The volatile oil consists of aplotaxen ($C_{17}H_{28}$), a-, b-costen ($C_{15}H_{24}$), costus acid ($C_{15}H_{22}O_3$), costus lactone ($C_{15}H_{20}O_2$), dihydrocostus lactone ($C_{15}H_{22}O_2$), costol ($C_{15}H_{24}O$) and small amounts of camphorene, phellandrene, etc. Traditionally, it is used mainly for improving the general health, in promoting digestion, and similar.

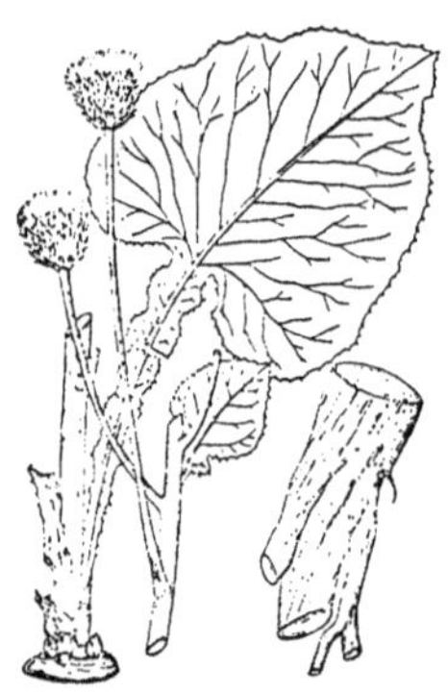

云木香

Fig. 39 Saussurea lappa Clarke (51)

Scutellaria baicalensis Georgi "Huang-chen" (9,11,39,51)

This herb, about 20-60 cm high, belongs to the Labiatae family. The root is used as medicine (Radix scutellariae). Its cross section has a needle-like appearance, dark yellow around the outer layers, brownish black in the center. It has no odor but a bitter taste. It contains baicalin and wogonin; the former is composed from baicalein with one molecule of glucuronic acid.

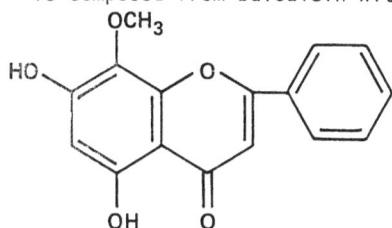

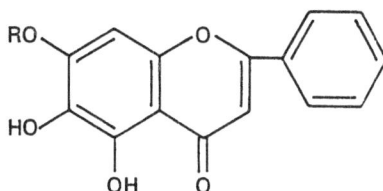

Wogonin

Baicalin (R = glucuronic acid)

Traditionally, it is used to reduce fever, as a diuretic agent, and to prevent miscarriage. Pharmacological tests have proved this herb effective in lowering blood pressure, elevating blood sugar level, and reducing fever with some anti-bacterial action. It also has an inhibiting action on the influenza virus. Clinically, it has been used to treat hypertension.

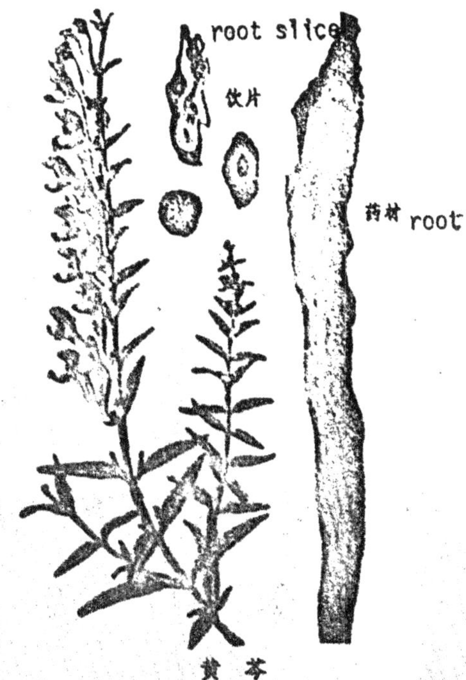

Fig. 40 Scutellaria baicalensis Georgi. (11)

Taraxacum mongolicum Hand.-Mazz. "Pu-kung-yin" or "Kung-yin" (11,15,30,39)

This herb is seen everywhere, is 10-25 cm tall, and belongs to the Compositae family. The whole plant, including root, is used as medicine. It contains taraxacin, taraxacerin, taraxasterol ($C_{29}H_{24}OH$), taraxerol, pectinum and choline, etc. Traditionally, it is used as a detoxifying agent, for swelling, and external wounds.

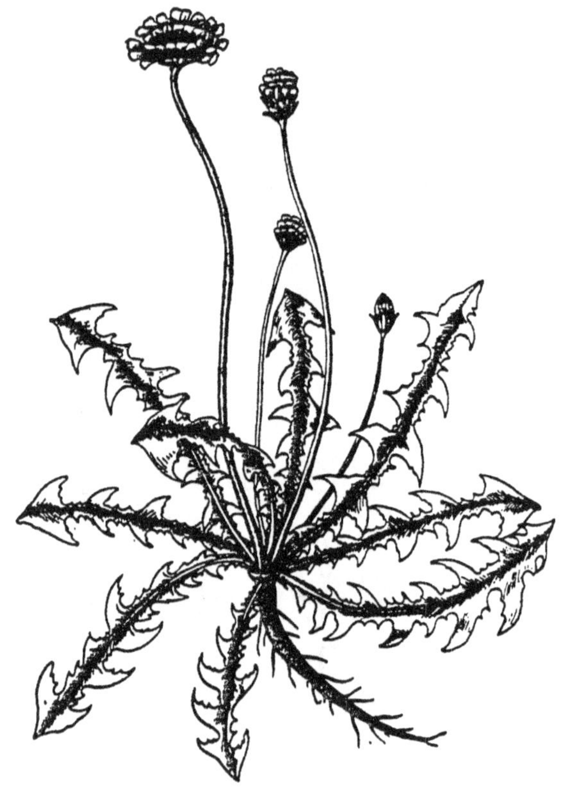

Fig. 41 Taraxacum mongolicum Hand. - Mazz. (11)

<u>Ulmus parvifolia Jacq.</u> "Lang-yu" (15,30)

This is a semi-evergreen tree with a height of about 20 m. It belongs to the <u>Urticaceae</u> family, and is widely grown on road sides, lake banks and in similar places. It tastes very bitter but contains no toxicity. It contains starch, tannin, ergosterol and other sterols. Traditionally, it is used mostly for external dressing on wounds and ulcerous tissues.

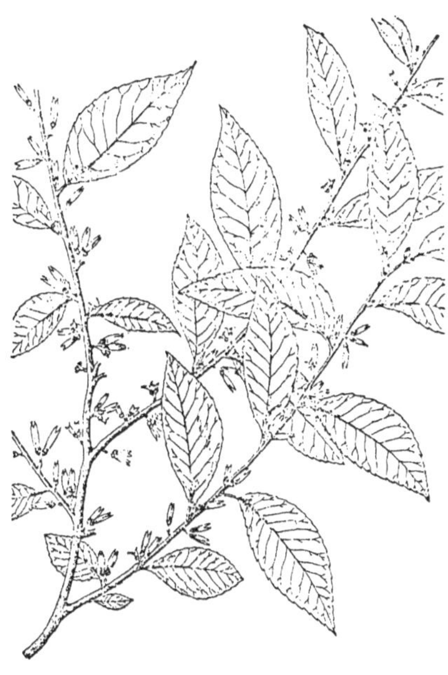

榔 榆

Fig. 42 <u>Ulmus parvifolia Jacq.</u> (30)

<u>Zingiber officinale Rosc.</u> "Chiang" or "Kan-chiang" (15,29,51)

This herb has a horizontal stem that grows underground; the stalk has a height of about 1 m. It belongs to the <u>Zingiberaceae</u> family. The underground stem is used as medicine (<u>Rhizoma zingiberis</u>), as well as a regular spice regularly used in oriental cooking. It contains 0.25 - 3 percent volatile oil, mainly zingiberol ($C_{15}H_{26}O$), zingiberene ($C_{15}H_{24}$), and camphorene. There are also small amounts of zingirol, resin and starch. The zingirol is a yellow oily liquid that tastes very hot. When this liquid, a mixture of zingerone and shogaol, is treated with 5 percent KOH solution, the hot taste is lost. Traditionally, it is used to reduce gas pain and other discomforts related to indigestion. It is also believed effective in treating roundworm. In some compound prescriptions, it is effective in stopping pain and in stopping bleeding.

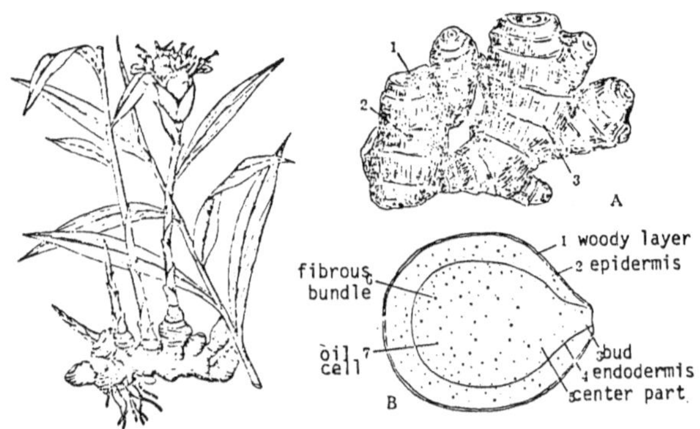

Fig. 43 <u>Zingiber officinale Rosc.</u> (51)

Zizyphus sativa var. spinosa (Bge.) "Suan-tsao-jen" (11,39,51)

This shrub or small tree grows in shady areas and widely distributed places and belongs to the Rhamnaceae family. The dried seeds, free from shells, are used as medicine (Semen zizyphi spinosae). It has no odor but tastes slightly bitter. The seed meal contains saponin, mainly composed from betulic acid ($C_{30}H_{48}O_3$) and betulin ($C_{30}H_{50}O_2$). There also are fatty oil, about 32 percent, protein, ergosterol, and some organic acids. Traditionally, it is an exellent tranquilizing agent. Clinical tests have shown this herb is effective in treating insomnia; the adult dose is 15 to 25 seeds (equivalent to 0.8 - 1.2 g). However, if the dosage increases to twice as much, it is poisonous; the patient may lose consciousness, lapsing into a coma. Based on pharmacological tests, this herb has a controlling effect on the central nervous system; it can create a calmed and hypnotized state. When over-processed to lose its oily appearance, it also loses its tranquilizing effect. It is speculated that the effective components are some of the water soluble organic compounds. In addition to the above-mentioned uses, it also can lower blood pressure, block heart conductivity, and stimulate the uterus.

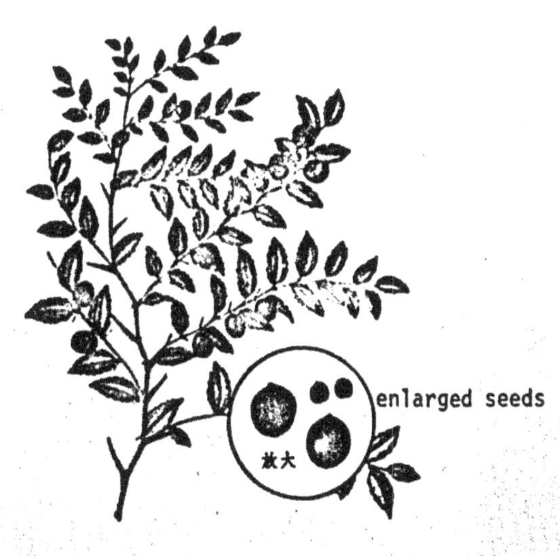

酸枣仁

Fig. 44 Zizyphus sativa var. spinosa (Bge.) (11)

CONCLUSION

Herbal medicine is believed to be an important component of Chinese traditional medicine. It is considered a well organized system of knowledge worked out by individual scholars as well as by governments in ancient times.

The first book on medicinal herbs was published approximately 2,000 years ago and has been revised and extended from time to time. An important revised edition was published in A.D. 659. The famed Li Shih-chen's work on the subject was published in 1578. There are many excellent drawings of herbs in Li's books.

When Western medicine was introduced into China in the nineteenth century, Chinese traditional medicine came to be regarded as unscientific and consequently was almost lost. However, with the founding of the People's Republic of China, it was revived and has since been regarded as a national treasure. The Chinese are now attempting to combine the two systems, traditional and Western, into one coherent entity. Various diseases are treated with a combination of both Western and traditional Chinese methods, including herbal drugs; this is the new medical trend in China. Some success has already been achieved, as is illustrated by the following:

1. The Chinese have since 1949 collected and identified more than 2,000 new medicinal herbs. Many clinically useful chemical compounds have been isolated from the herbs and some of the compounds have been synthesized.

2. Ancient medical theories are being applied clinically in the light of modern sciences. For instance, acute appendicitis and gallstones have reportedly been treated successfully with herbal medicine without surgery.

3. A number of single herbs and mixtures of herbs have been developed for the treatment of coronary diseases. Some of these are claimed to be very effective.

4. The Chinese are now using herbs in conjunction with Western medicine for cancer therapy. The Chinese believe that certain herbs have a beneficial effect on cancer patients by improving their general health and by stimulating their appetite. Whether the herbs can stimulate immunity against cancer cells and increase the patient's tolerance for the common Western anti-cancer drugs is not yet known.

The blending of Chinese traditional medicine with Western science potentially could have great influence on the future development of Western medicine.

REFERENCES

1. Ansan shih shu kuang Mao-che-tung ssu hsiang liao hsuan chuan tsu, ed. Treatment of Rheumatic Heart Disease by the Combination of Western and Chinese Traditional Medicine. (Chung Hsi I Chieh Ho Chih Liao Feng Szu Hsing Hsin Tsang Pin Ti Ti Hui), People's Public Health Publisher, Peking, 1972.

2. "Back to folk medicine: the pros and cons," Medical World News, pp.65-68, 1973.

3. Chekiang shen wei sheng chu, ed. Traditionally Used Chinese Materia Medica in Chekiang, No. III, (Chekiang Min Chien Chang Yung Tsao Yao, No. III), Chekiang People's Publisher, Hanchou, 1972.

4. Chen, Hsin-chien. Newly Edited Materia Medica, (Hsin Pien Yao Wu Hsueh). Commercial Press, Hongkong, 1971.

5. "The Chinese Medicinal Herbs," (a motion picture), The China Film Distribution and Exhibition Corp., Peking, 1973.

6. Chu Santung i hsueh yuan kung chun hsuan tui and Santung i hsueh yuan ko ming wei yuan hui, ed. Handbook of Materia Medica, (Yao Wu Shou Tze), Shantung People's Publisher, 1971.

7. Chu, Chen-poh, ed. Newly Edited Chinese Materia Medica, (Chung Yao Hsin Pien), Tai-ping Publisher, Hongkong, 1968.

8. Chung i yen chiu Kuang-an-men i yuan, ed. Combined Traditional and Western Medicine in Treating Rectum and Colon Disorders, (Chung Hsi I Chien Ho Chih Liao Kang Men Chih Chang Chi Ping), People's Publisher, Peking, 1972.

9. Chung i yen chiu yuan chung yao yen chiu ssu, ed. "Studies on the chemical constituents of traditional drug Scutellaria baicalensis (Huang-chen)," Chin.med.J., 7:417-420, 1973

10. Chung kuo i hsueh ko hsueh yuan and Yao wu yen chiu so ko ming wei yuan hui, ed. Handbook on Cultivation of Commonly Used Chinese Materia Medica, (Chang Yung Chung Tsao Yao Tsai Pei Shou Tze), People's Public Health Publisher, Peking, 1971.

11. Chung kuo i hsueh ko hsueh yuan yao wu yen chiu so ko ming wei yuan hui and Chekiang chung i hsueh yuan ko ming wei yuan hui, ed. Atlas of Commonly Used Chinese Materia Medica, (Chang Yung Chung Tsao Yao Tu Pu), People's Public Health Publisher, Peking, 1970.

12. Chung kuo i hsueh ko hsueh yuan yao wu yen chiu so yao li shih et al, ed. "Absorption, distribution and excretion of anisodamine," Chin.med.J., 5:275-278, 1973.

13. Chung kuo i hsueh ko hsueh yuan yao wu yen chiu so yao li shih et al, ed. "Pharmacologic effects of anisodamine," Chin.med.J., 5:269-273, 1973.

14. Chung kuo i hsueh ko hsueh yuan yao wu yen chiu so, ed. Lin-chih, (Fomes japonicus Fr.), People's Publisher, Peking, 1973.

15. Chung kuo i hsueh ko hsueh yuan yao wu yen chiu tsu, ed. Studies of Effective Components in Chinese Herbal Medicine I, (Chung Tsao Yao Yu Hsiao Chen Fen Ti Yen Chiu I), People's Public Health Publisher, Peking, 1972.

16. Chung kuo i hsueh ko hsueh yuan yao wu yen chiu tsu, ed. Studies of Effective Components in Chinese Herbal Medicine II, (Chung Tsao Yao Yu Hsiao Chen Fen Ti Yen Chiu II), People's Public Health Publisher, Peking, 1972.

17. Chung kuo i hsueh ko hsueh yuan, ed. Handbook of Drug Therapy, (Yao Wu Chih Liao Shou Tze), People's Public Health Publisher, 1970.

18. Chung kuo jen ming chieh fang chun ti shih liu shih i pu tui wei sheng tui, ed. "Burns treated principally with traditional herb medicine," Chin.med.J., 8:497-498, 1973.

19. Chung kuo ko hsueh yuan hua nan tze wu yen chiu tsu, ed. Atlas of Commonly Used Chinese Materia Medica in Color, No. I, (Chang Yung Chung Tsao Yao Tsai Shih Tu Pu), Kuang-tung People's Publisher, Canton, 1970.

20. Chung san i hsueh yuan, "Treatment of 103 cases of coronary diseases with Ilex pubescens Hook. et Arn., Chin. med.J., 1:64, 1973.

21. Chung, Yong. Food as Medicine, V. I & II, (Shi Liao Yao Wu, V. I & II), Te-li Bookstore, Hongkong, 1972.

22. "Combined Tang-seng extract for coronary diseases," Chin.med.J., 6:330, 1973.

23. Handbook of Commonly Used Chinese Materia Medica, (Chang Yung Chung Tsao Yao Shou Tze), Commercial Press, Hongkong, 1970.

24. Honan shen lo yang shih ti san jen ming i yuan chuan jan ping ko, ed. "Anisodamine in treatment of severe toxic bacillary dysentery," Chin.med.J., 8:492-493, 1973.

25. Hopeh chung i yen chiu yuan, ed. Selected Prescriptions of Chinese Traditional Internal Medicine, (Chung I Nei Ko Yen Fang Kuo Hsuan), Commercial Press, Hongkong, 1971.

26. Hopeh shen ko ming wei yuan hui shang yeh chu i yao kung yin chan et al. ed. Handbook of Chinese Materia Medica in Hopeh, (Hopeh Chung Yao Shou Tze), Science Publisher, 1970.

27. Hsitsang tzu chih chu ko ming wei yuan hui wei sheng chu and Hsitsang chun chu hou chin pu wei sheng shu, ed. Commonly Used Chinese Materia Medica in Hsitsang, (Hsitsang Chang Yung Chung Tsao Yao), Hsitsang People's Publisher, 1971.

28. Hunan chung i hsueh yuan, ed. Clinical Handbook of Commonly Used Herbal Medicines, (Lin Chuang Chang Yung Chung Yao Shou Tze), People's Public Health Publisher, Peking, 1972.

29. Hunan chung i yao yen chiu tsu, ed. Hunan Materia Medica I, (Hunan Yao Wu Tze I), Hunan People's Publisher, Changsha, 1970.

30. Hunan chung i yao yen chiu tsu, ed. Hunan Materia Medica II, (Hunan Yao Wu Tze II), Hunan People's Publisher, Changsha, 1972.

31. Kansu ko ming wei yuan hui wei sheng chu, ed. An Introduction to Chinese Traditional Medicine, (Hsin Pien Chung I Ju Men), Kansu People's Publisher, 1970.

32. Kansu shen ko ming wei yuan hui wei sheng chu, ed. Handbook of Chinese Materia Medica in Kansu, No. II, (Kansu Chung Tsao Yao Shou Tze, No. II), Kansu People's Publisher, 1971.

33. Kao, J.C. "Research on Chinese traditional herbal medicine since liberation," Journal of Chinese Traditional Medicine, 8:315-320, 1963.

34. Kiangsu hsin i hsueh yuan. Chinese Traditional Medicine, (Chung I Hsueh), Kiangsu People's Publisher, 1972.

35. Kirin shen sheng pien hsi hsiao tsu, ed. Diagnosis, Treatment, and Prevention of Tumors, (Chung Liu Ti Chen Tuan Yu Fang Chih), Kirin People's Publisher, 1973.

36. Koo, W.Y. A Report on the Studies of Chinese Drugs, School of Pharmacy, National Taiwan University, Taiwan, 1967.

37. Kuang-An-Men Chinese Traditional Hospital, Peking, The author's personal observation, 1973.

38. Kuangchou chungsan i hsueh yuan chung liu i yuan, ed. The Prevention and Treatment of Common Tumors, (Chang Chien Chung Liu Ti Fang Chih), Canton People's Publisher, 1972.

39. Kuangchou pu tui hou chin pu wei sheng pu tsu tzu. Newly Edited Outline of Chinese Traditional Medicine, (Hsin Pien Chung I Hsueh Chai Yao), People's Public Health Publisher, Peking, 1973.

40. Kuanghsi tu tsu tzu chih chu ko ming wei yuan hui wei sheng kuan li fu wu chan, ed. Chinese Materia Medica in Kuanghsi No. II, (Kuanghsi Chung Tsao Yao No. II), Kuanghsi People's Publisher, 1970.

41. Kuangtung chung i hsueh yuan. Newly Edited Chinese Traditional Medicine, (Hsin Pien Chung I Hsueh), Shanghai People's Publisher, Shanghai, 1971.

42. Kuangtung chung i hsueh yuan. An Introductory Note to Medicine, (Tan Tan Tsu Kuo I Hsueh), Kuangtung People's Publisher, 1972.

43. Kuei-chou shen chung i yen chiu so, ed. Kuei-chou Materia Medica, No. II, (Kuei-chou Tsao Yao, NO. II), Kuei-chou People's Publisher, 1970.

44. Kuei-chou shen chung i yen chiu so, ed. Kuei-chou Materia Medica, No. III, (Kuei-chou Tsao Yao, No. III), Kuei-chou People's Publisher, 1970.

45. Li, bin. Tumor Institute and Hospital, Peking, Personal Communication, 1973.

46. Li, C.P. "An introduction note to ginseng," The American Journal of Chinese Medicine, V. 1, No. 2:249-261, 1973.

47. Li, C.P. Anticancer agents in the People's Republic of China, Fogarty International Center, U.S. National Institutes of Health, Bethesda, Maryland, 1974.

48. Lin, Wen-kuang. Treatment of Snakebite, (Tu She Yao Shang Fang Chih Fa), Hung-yeh Medical Publisher, Hongkong, 1971.

49. Liu, S.S. Abstracts on the Research of Traditional Medicine, 1820-1961, Science Publisher, Peking, 1965.

50. Liu, S.S. Abstracts on the Research of Traditional Medicine, 2nd. ed., pp.894, 1971. Science Publisher, Peking

51. Lou, T.C., ed. Pharmacognosy, (Sheng Yao Hsueh), People's Public Health Publisher, Peking, 1965.

52. Lucas, R., Nature's Medicines, Wilshire Book Co., California, 1972.

53. Meng, C.W., "Several steps of medical progress in China," Scientia, 11:324-328, 1957.

54. Nantung i hsueh yuan fu shu i yuan shao shang hsiao tsu, ed. "Clinical application of Ilex chinensis Sims (Shih-chi ching) in treatment of burns," Chin.med.J., 4:217-220, 1973.

55. Nei meng ko tzu chih chu ko ming wei yuan hui wei sheng chu, ed. Chinese Materia Medica in Inner Mongolia, (Nei Meng Ko Chung Tsao Yao), Inner Mongolia Publisher, 1972.

56. Peking pu tui hou pu wei sheng pu et al, ed. Handbook of Commonly Used Chinese Materia Medica in Northern China, (Pei Fang Chang Yung Chung Tsao Yao Shou Tze), People's Public Health Publisher, Peking, 1971.

57. Peking shih chung i i yuan, ed. Differential Diagnosis and Appropriate Treatment, (Pien Cheng Shih Chih Kang Yao), People's Publisher, Peking, 1973.

58. Peking yu yi i yuan er ko et al, ed. "Anisodamine therapy of diseases of acute microcirculatory disturbances," Chin.med.J., 5:259-263, 1973.

59. "Pharmacological studies of Ilex chinensis Sims," Chin.med.J., 4:204, 1973.

60. Santung* chung tsao yao shou tze pien hsi hsiao tsu, ed. Handbook of Chinese Materia Medica in Santung, (Santung Chung Tsao Yao Shou Tze), Santung People's Publisher, 1970.

61. Shanghai chang yung chung tsao yao pien hsi tsu, ed. Commonly Used Chinese Materia Medica in Shanghai, (Shanghai Chang Yung Chung Tsao Yao), Shanghai Municipal Publisher, Shanghai, 1970.

62. Shanghai chung i hsueh yuan. Differential Diagnosis and Appropriate Treatment, (Pien Cheng Shih Chih), Shanghai People's Publisher, Shanghai, 1972.

63. Shanghai Chung i hsueh yuan, ed. Handbook of Chinese Traditional Prescriptions for Clinical Use, (Chung I Fang Chi Lin Chuang Shou Tze), Shanghai People's Publisher, 1973.

*Can also be spelled as Shantung.

64. Shanghai Institute of Hypertension, "Experimental studies on the mechanism of action of some traditional Chinese compound prescriptions which are effective in the treatment of hypertension," Zhong Neike Z, 9:12, 1961.

65. Shanghai ti er i hsueh yuan fu shu jui king i yuan shao shang ko and Shanghai chung yao chih yao san chang, ed. "Clinical observations on action of ointment Yuchuang No. 10 in separation of eschars," Chin.med.J., 4:226-228, 1973.

66. Shanghai ti i i hsueh yuan hua san i yuan, ed. "Acute myocardial infarction treated with traditional and Western medicine," Chin.med.J., 129-32, 1973.

67. Shensi chung i fu shu i yuan wai ko. "Combined traditional and Western medicine in 134 cases of acute abdominal conditions." Shensi New Medicine, 1-2:27-36, 1973

68. Shensi shen ko ming wei yuan hiu wei sheng chu and shang yeh chu, ed. Chinese Materia Medica in Shensi, (Shensi Chung Tsao Yao), Science Publisher, 1971.

69. Tai, Kan-lin. The Technology of Chinese Traditional Pharmaceuticals, (Ying-hsiao-kao-tan-wan-san Chih Fa), Te-li Bookstore, Hongkong, 1971.

70. "Three varieties of Aquifoliaceae family herbs," Chin. med.J., 3:150, 1973.

71. Tientsin chung i hsueh yuan, ed. Clinical Handbook of Chinese Traditional Medicine, (Chung I Shih Yung Lin Chuang Shou Tze), Shang-wu Publisher, Shanghai, 1970.

72. Tientsin shih nan kai i yuan, ed. "Combined traditional and Western medicine in acute abdominal conditions," Chin. med.J., 1:33-39, 1973.

73. Tsun-yi i hsueh yuan ko ming wei yuan hui, ed. Combined Traditional and Western Medicine in Acute Abdominal Conditions, (Chung Hsi I Chieh Ho Chih Liao Chi Fu Cheng), People's Public Health Publisher, Peking, 1972.

74. Tung, Cheng-lung and Tao, Shou-chi, ed. Practical Cardiology, (Shih Yung Hsin Tsang Ping Hsueh), Shanghai People's Publisher, Shanghai, 1960.

75. Yi Ning-yu, et al. "Pharmacologic studies on Liu Wei Di Huang T'ang (Decoction of Rehmannia with 6 components) - its action on kidney function and blood pressure of rats with renal hypertension" Chin.med.J., 84:433-436, 1965.

76. Yunnan shen wei sheng chu ko ming wei yuan hui, ed. Chinese Materia Medica in Yunnan, (Yunnan Chung Tsao Yao), Yunnan People's Publisher, Kunming, 1971.

ACKNOWLEDGEMENTS

The author wishes to express his gratitude to Dr. D.C. Dju Chang for her excellent assistance in the development of this monograph. He is also grateful to Mrs. Lotta Chi and Mrs. Ruth Cheng Li for their valuable assistance.

During the author's trip to China in July and August, 1973, his wife, Dr. H.C. Tang, helped to interview the Chinese biomedical scientists, examined patients in hospitals, and analyzed clinical information. The author's nephew, Prof. C.W. Li, purchased for the author approximately 60 biomedical reference books and a number of rare herbal specimens in different cities. Both Dr. Tang and Prof. Li took careful notes during the author's visit to various medical institutions and hospitals. Their work was a very valuable aid in the preparation of this monograph.

Finally, my thanks are due to the Fogarty International Center, National Institutes of Health, Bethesda, Maryland for its publication of this monograph as well as its support of my travel to the People's Republic of China.

PARTICIPANTS IN THE PREPARATION OF THIS MONOGRAPH

Li, C.P., M.D. Former chief, Virus Biology Section, LVR., D.B.S., National Institutes of Health, Bethesda, Maryland. Author of _Anticancer Agents in People's Republic of China_, Fogarty International Center, N.I.H.

Chang, Dsai-Chwen Dju, Ph.D. (biochemistry) Former Professor of National Taiwan University, Taiwan.

Tang, Han-Chih, M.D. Internist in geriatrics and cardiology, St. Elizabeth's Hospital, Washington, D.C.

Showell, John S., Ph.D. (organic chemistry) Program Director in Organic and Synthetic Chemistry, National Science Foundation.

Chi, Lotta Li, M.S. (bacteriology)

Ruth Cheng Li, M.S. (microbiology)

Showell, Ellen H., B.A. (English)

INDEX

A

A (continued)

B

B (continued)

C

C (continued)

D

D (continued)

E

F

G

G (continued)

M

N

O

P

R

R (continued)

S

S (continued)

T

U

V

W

X

Z

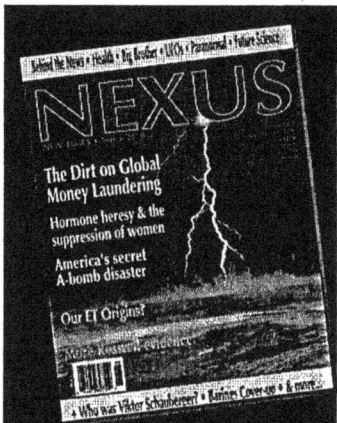

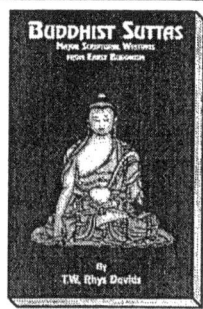

www.ingramcontent.com/pod-product-compliance
Lightning Source LLC
Chambersburg PA
CBHW030022290326
41934CB00005B/440
9781585092192